This report contains the collective views of an international group of experts and does not necessarily represent the decisions or the stated policy of the United Nations Environment Programme, the International Labour Organisation, or the World Health Organization.

Environmental Health Criteria 114

DIMETHYLFORMAMIDE

Published under the joint sponsorship of
the United Nations Environment Programme,
the International Labour Organisation,
and the World Health Organization

First draft prepared by Dr A. Bainova,
Institute of Hygeine and Occupational Health, Sofia, Bulgaria

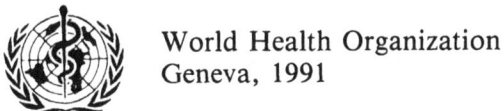

World Health Organization
Geneva, 1991

The International Programme on Chemical Safety (IPCS) is a joint venture of the United Nations Environment Programme, the International Labour Organisation, and the World Health Organization. The main objective of the IPCS is to carry out and disseminate evaluations of the effects of chemicals on human health and the quality of the environment. Supporting activities include the development of epidemiological, experimental laboratory, and risk-assessment methods that could produce internationally comparable results, and the development of manpower in the field of toxicology. Other activities carried out by the IPCS include the development of know-how for coping with chemical accidents, coordination of laboratory testing and epidemiological studies, and promotion of research on the mechanisms of the biological action of chemicals.

WHO Library Cataloguing in Publication Data

Dimethylformamide

(Environmental health criteria ; 114)

1.Dimethylformamide - adverse effects 2.Dimethylformamide - toxicity
I.Series

ISBN 92 4 157114 4   (NLM Classification: QV 633)
ISSN 0250-863X

© World Health Organization 1991

Publications of the World Health Organization enjoy copyright protection in accordance with the provisions of Protocol 2 of the Universal Copyright Convention. For rights of reproduction or translation of WHO publications, in part or *in toto*, application should be made to the Office of Publications, World Health Organization, Geneva, Switzerland. The World Health Organization welcomes such applications.

The designations employed and the presentation of the material in this publication do not imply the expression of any opinion whatsoever on the part of the Secretariat of the World Health Organization concerning the legal status of any country, territory, city or area or of its authorities, or concerning the delimitation of its frontiers or boundaries.

The mention of specific companies or of certain manufacturers' products does not imply that they are endorsed or recommended by the World Health Organization in preference to others of a similar nature that are not mentioned. Errors and omissions excepted, the names of proprietary products are distinguished by initial capital letters.

PRINTED IN FINLAND
Vammalan Kirjapaino Oy
91/8803 — VAMMALA — 5000

CONTENTS

ENVIRONMENTAL HEALTH CRITERIA FOR
DIMETHYLFORMAMIDE

	Page
1. SUMMARY AND EVALUATION, CONCLUSIONS, RECOMMENDATIONS	11
1.1 Summary and evaluation	11
1.1.1 General properties	11
1.1.2 Environmental transport, distribution, and transformation	11
1.1.3 Environmental levels and human exposure	11
1.1.4 Kinetics and metabolism	12
1.1.5 Effects on organisms in the environment	12
1.1.6 Effects on experimental animals and *in vitro* test systems	12
1.1.7 Effects on human beings	13
1.2 Conclusions	14
1.3 Recommendations	15
1.3.1 Safe handling	15
1.3.2 Further research	15
2. IDENTITY, PHYSICAL AND CHEMICAL PROPERTIES, ANALYTICAL METHODS	16
2.1 Identity	16
2.2 Physical and chemical properties	16
2.3 Organoleptic properties	18
2.4 Analytical methods	18
2.4.1 Determination of DMF in workplace air	18
2.4.2 Determination of DMF and metabolites in biological media	18
2.4.3 Determination of DMF in soil, plants, and food	19

	Page
3. SOURCES OF HUMAN AND ENVIRONMENTAL EXPOSURE	21
3.1 Natural occurrence	21
3.2 Man-made sources	21
3.2.1 Production and uses	21
3.2.1.1 Production	21
3.2.1.2 Uses	22
4. ENVIRONMENTAL TRANSPORT, DISTRIBUTION, AND TRANSFORMATION	24
4.1 Transport and distribution between media	24
4.1.1 Air	24
4.1.2 Water	24
4.1.3 Soil	25
4.1.4 Bioaccumulation	26
5. ENVIRONMENTAL LEVELS AND HUMAN EXPOSURE	27
5.1 Environmental levels	27
5.1.1 Air	27
5.1.2 Water	27
5.1.3 Soil	28
5.2 General population exposure	28
5.3 Occupational exposure	28
5.3.1 Concentrations in the workplace air	28
5.3.2 Dermal exposure	30
6. KINETICS AND METABOLISM	32
6.1 Animal studies	32
6.1.1 Absorption	32
6.1.2 Distribution	32
6.1.3 Metabolic transformation	34
6.1.4 Elimination and excretion	39
6.1.5 Metabolic interaction between DMF and ethanol	40

			Page
6.2	Human studies		43
	6.2.1	Absorption, distribution, metabolism, excretion	43
	6.2.2	The influence of ethanol on DMF metabolism in human volunteers	44
	6.2.3	Biological monitoring of workers	44
		6.2.3.1 Determination of NMF in the urine	44
		6.2.3.2 N,N-dimethylformamide determination in the expired air	48
		6.2.3.3 Appraisal	49
7.	EFFECTS ON ORGANISMS IN THE ENVIRONMENT		50
8.	EFFECTS ON EXPERIMENTAL ANIMALS AND *IN VITRO* TEST SYSTEMS		52
8.1	Single exposures		52
8.2	Skin and eye irritation, sensitization		52
	8.2.1	Skin irritation	52
	8.2.2	Eye irritation	55
	8.2.3	Sensitization	55
8.3	Repeated exposure		56
8.4	Specific organ toxicity		56
	8.4.1	Liver	56
	8.4.2	Gastrointestinal tract	63
	8.4.3	Cardiovascular system	63
	8.4.4	Kidney	63
	8.4.5	Nervous system	64
	8.4.6	Lungs	65
	8.4.7	Haematopoietic system	65
	8.4.8	Adrenals	66
	8.4.9	Gonads	66
8.5	Developmental toxicity and reproduction		66
	8.5.1	Developmental toxicity	74
		8.5.1.1 Mouse	74
		8.5.1.2 Rat	74
		8.5.1.3 Rabbit	77
		8.5.1.4 Appraisal	79

		Page
8.6	Mutagenicity and related end-points	79
	8.6.1 *In vitro* studies	78
	8.6.2 *In vivo* studies	83
	8.6.3 Appraisal	83
8.7	Carcinogenicity	85
8.8	Induction of tumour cell differentiation	85
8.9	Mechanism of toxicity, mode of action	86

9. EFFECTS ON HUMAN BEINGS 87

9.1	General population exposure	87
9.2	Occupational exposure	87
	9.2.1 Accidental poisoning	87
	9.2.2 Long-term exposure	87
	9.2.3 Epidemiological studies on carcinogenicity	88
	9.2.4 Alcohol intolerance	95

10. PREVIOUS EVALUATIONS BY INTERNATIONAL BODIES 96

REFERENCES 97

RESUME ET EVALUATION, CONCLUSIONS, RECOMMANDATIONS 113

RESUMEN Y EVALUACION, CONCLUSIONES, RECOMENDACIONES 119

TASK GROUP MEETING ON ENVIRONMENTAL HEALTH CRITERIA FOR DIMETHYLFORMAMIDE

Members

Dr A. Aitio, International Agency for Research on Cancer, World Health Organization, Lyon, France (*Chairman*)

Dr A. Bainova, Institute of Hygiene and Occupational Health, Sofia, Bulgaria (*Co-rapporteur*)

Ms J. Favilla, Office of Toxic Substances, US Environmental Protection Agency, Washington, USA

Dr G.L. Kennedy, Jr, Haskell Laboratory for Toxicology and Industrial Medicine, EI du Pont de Nemours & Co., Newark, Delaware, USA (*Co-rapporteur*)

Professor N.P. Misra, Department of Medicine, Gandhi Medical College, Bhopal, India

Dr K. Morimoto, Division of Medical Chemistry, National Institute of Hygienic Sciences, Tokyo, Japan (*Vice-Chairman*)

Dr C. Sadarangani, Petrochemical Industries Co. (KSC), Ahmadi, Kuwait

Dr V. Scailteur, Procter and Gamble GmbH, Frankfurt, Germany

Dr Yu Hui Qin, Institute of Environmental Health Monitoring, Chinese Academy of Preventive Medicine, Beijing, China

Observers

Dr R. Jäckh, European Chemical Industries Ecology and Toxicology Centre, Brussels, Belgium

Secretariat

Dr R. Hertel, Fraunhofer Institute for Toxicology and Aerosol Research, Hanover, Federal Republic of Germany

Dr K.W. Jager, International Programme on Chemical Safety, World Health Organization, Geneva, Switzerland (*Secretary*)

Dr P.G. Jenkins, International Programme on Chemical Safety, World Health Organization, Geneva, Switzerland

NOTE TO READERS OF THE CRITERIA DOCUMENTS

Every effort has been made to present information in the criteria documents as accurately as possible without unduly delaying their publication. In the interest of all users of the environmental health criteria documents, readers are kindly requested to communicate any errors that may have occurred to the Manager of the International Programme on Chemical Safety, World Health Organization, Geneva, Switzerland, in order that they may be included in corrigenda, which will appear in subsequent volumes.

* * *

A detailed data profile and a legal file can be obtained from the International Register of Potentially Toxic Chemicals, Palais des Nations, 1211 Geneva 10, Switzerland (Telephone no. 7988400 - 7985850).

ENVIRONMENTAL HEALTH CRITERIA FOR DIMETHYLFORMAMIDE

A WHO Task Group on Environmental Health Criteria for Dimethylformamide, which met in Wolfsburg from 13 to 17 March 1989, was organized by the Fraunhofer Institute for Toxicology and Aerosol Research, Hanover, Federal Republic of Germany. The meeting was sponsored by the Federal Government. Dr K.W. Jager of the IPCS opened the meeting and welcomed the participants on behalf of the three cooperating organizations of the IPCS (UNEP/ILO/WHO). The Task Group reviewed and revised the draft criteria document and made an evaluation of the risks for human health and the environment from exposure to dimethylformamide.

The first and second drafts of this document were prepared by Dr A. BAINOVA of the Institute of Hygiene and Occupational Health, Sofia, Bulgaria. Dr K.W. JAGER of the Central Unit, International Programme on Chemical Safety, was responsible for the scientific content of the document and Mrs M.O. HEAD of Oxford for the editing.

The efforts of all who helped in the preparation and finalization of the document are gratefully acknowledged.

1. SUMMARY AND EVALUATION, CONCLUSIONS, RECOMMENDATIONS

1.1 Summary and evaluation

1.1.1 General properties

N,N-dimethylformamide (dimethylformamide, DMF, CAS 68-12-2) is an organic solvent produced in large quantities throughout the world. It is used in the chemical industry as a solvent, an intermediate, and an additive. DMF is a colourless liquid with an unpleasant slight odour that, nevertheless, has poor warning properties. It is usually stable but, when it comes in contact with strong oxidizers, halogens, alkylaluminium, or halogenated hydrocarbons (especially in combination with metals), it may cause fires and explosions. DMF is completely miscible with water and most organic solvents. It has a relatively low vapour pressure.

Gas chromatographic procedures for determining DMF are available.

1.1.2 Environmental transport, distribution, and transformation

DMF is stable in ambient air, but may undergo microbial and algal degradation in water. Adapted microorganisms and activated sludge efficiently biodegrade DMF. As a result of its complete solubility in water, DMF moves readily through soils and would not be expected to accumulate in the food chain.

1.1.3 Environmental levels and human exposure

DMF does not occur naturally. There are few data concerning environmental levels or the exposure of the general population to DMF. Concentrations in the air in the range of 0.02-0.12 mg/m^3 have been found in residential areas, near industrial sites. DMF has rarely been detected in the water of heavily industrialized river basins, and then only at concentrations below 0.01 mg/litre.

Data are not available on the levels of DMF in soil, plants, wildlife, and food.

Summary

Occupational exposure occurs via skin contact with DMF liquid and vapour, and through the inhalation of vapour. Concentrations of 3-86 mg/m^3 air have been detected, with peaks of up to 600 mg/m^3, during the repair or maintenance of machines. In a few unusual situations, levels of up to 4500 mg/m^3 have been reported.

1.1.4 Kinetics and metabolism

Toxic amounts of DMF may be absorbed by inhalation and through the skin. Absorbed DMF is distributed uniformly. The metabolic transformation of DMF takes place mainly in the liver, with the aid of microsomal enzyme systems. In animals and human beings, the main product of DMF biotransformation is *N*-hydroxymethyl-*N*-methylformamide (DMF-OH). This metabolite is converted during gas chromatographic analysis to *N*-methylformamide, which is itself (together with *N*-hydroxy methylformamide and formamide) a minor metabolite. Thus, in metabolic studies and biological monitoring, urinary concentrations of metabolites are measured and expressed as NMF, though DMF-OH is the major contributor to this concentration. The determination of NMF/DMF-OH in the urine may be a suitable biological indicator of total DMF exposure.

In experimental animals, it has been demonstrated that DMF metabolism is saturated at high exposure levels and, at very high levels, DMF inhibits its own metabolism.

Metabolic interaction occurs between DMF and ethanol.

1.1.5 Effects on organisms in the environment

The effects of DMF on the environment have not been well studied. The toxicity for aquatic organisms appears to be low.

1.1.6 Effects on experimental animals and in vitro test systems

The acute toxicity of DMF in a variety of species is low (in rats, the oral LD_{50} is approximately 3000 mg/kg, the dermal LD_{50}, approximately 5000 mg/kg, and the inhalational LC_{50}, approximately 10 000 mg/m^3). It is a slight to moderate skin and eye irritant. One study on guinea-pigs indicated no sensitization potential. DMF can facilitate the absorption of other chemical substances through the skin.

Exposure of experimental animals to DMF via all routes of exposure may cause dose-related liver injury. Regeneration, after exposure has ceased, has been demonstrated. In some studies, signs of toxicity in the myocardium and kidneys have also been described.

DMF has not been shown to be toxic to the testes or ovaries of rats and effects on fertility have not been demonstrated. DMF has been found to be embryotoxic and a weak teratogen in rats, mice, and rabbits. The rabbit was found to be the most sensitive species when exposed via inhalation: teratogenic effects were observed at 1350 mg/m^3 (450 ppm) and above, but not at 450 mg/m^3 (150 ppm). After dermal exposure, a very low incidence of embryotoxic and teratogenic effects was observed in some studies at dose levels of between 100 and 400 mg/kg per day.

DMF was generally found to be inactive, both *in vitro* and *in vivo*, in an extensive set of short-term tests for genetic and related effects.

No adequate long-term carcinogenicity studies on experimental animals have been reported.

1.1.7 Effects on human beings

No adverse effects of DMF on the general population have been clearly demonstrated.

Skin irritation and conjunctivitis have been reported after direct contact with DMF.

After accidental exposure to high levels of DMF, abdominal pain, nausea, vomiting, dizziness, and fatigue occur within 48 h. Liver function may be disturbed, and blood pressure changes, tachycardia, and ECG abnormalities have been reported. Recovery is usually complete.

Following long-term repeated exposure, symptoms include headache, loss of appetite, and fatigue. Biochemical signs of liver dysfunction may be observed. Liver damage seems to occur only when the DMF exposure level exceeds 30 mg/m^3, in the absence of skin contact. This airborne level corresponds to approximately 40 mg NMF/DMF-OH/g creatinine in a post-shift urine sample.

Exposure to DMF, even at concentrations below 30 mg/m^3, may cause alcohol intolerance. Symptoms may include a sudden facial flush, tightness in the chest, and dizziness, sometimes accompanied by nausea and dyspnoea. They last from 2 to 4 h and disappear without treatment.

There is limited evidence that DMF is carcinogenic for human beings. An increased incidence of testicular tumours was reported in one study, whereas another study showed an increased incidence of tumours of the buccal cavity and pharynx, but not of the testes.

In two studies, which provide few details, an increased frequency of miscarriages was reported in women exposed to DMF, among other chemicals.

1.2. Conclusions

1. In view of the present uses of DMF, general population exposure is probably very low.

2. DMF is readily absorbed through the skin as well as via inhalation. Determination of urinary NMF/DMF-OH is a useful means of estimating the total amount of DMF absorbed.

3. The risk of liver damage is low, when the level of DMF in ambient air is kept below 30 mg/m^3 and there is no skin contact. A tentative value for the corresponding urinary NMF/DMF-OH level in a post-shift sample is 40 mg/g creatinine.

4. DMF is embryotoxic and a weak teratogen in rats, mice, and rabbits.

5. There is limited evidence of carcinogenicity of DMF for human beings.

6. Available data indicate low environmental toxicity. It is unlikely that bioaccumulation takes place.

1.3 Recommendations

1.3.1 Safe handling

1. Airborne concentrations should be maintained below 30 mg/m^3 and skin contact should be prevented.

2. Urinary NMF/DMF-OH, as an index of total exposure, should be monitored and maintained below 40 mg NMF/g creatinine in post-shift samples. If this level is exceeded, action should be taken to reduce exposure.

1.3.2 Further research

1. The possible carcinogenic effects of DMF in human beings should be investigated by means of studies on experimental animals and human populations.

2. More information is needed on the extrapolation of the embryotoxicity and teratogenicity of DMF from animal studies to human beings. Comparison of the kinetics of DMF in human beings and animals would be valuable.

3. There is a need for more information on the mechanisms of action and the relative potency of the metabolites of DMF in both animals and human beings.

4. The relationships should be refined between: (a) urinary metabolite concentrations and atmospheric exposure levels (in the absence of skin contact), and (b) total dose via all routes (as indicated by post-shift urinary NMF levels) and the absence of hepatotoxicity.

2. IDENTITY, PHYSICAL AND CHEMICAL PROPERTIES, ANALYTICAL METHODS

2.1 Identity

Chemical structure:	H₃C–N(–CH₃)–C(=O)H
Chemical formula:	C_3H_7NO
Common name:	dimethylformamide
Common synonyms:	N,N-dimethylformamide, DMF, DMFA, formdimethylamide
CAS registry number:	68-12-2
Relative molecular mass	73.1
Conversion factors: (at 20 °C)	1 ppm = 3 mg/m³ 1 mg/m³ = 0.33 ppm

2.2 Physical and chemical properties

Some physical properties of DMF (Eberling, 1980) are given in Table 1. DMF is a colourless, organic solvent, free from suspended matter. Technical DMF may contain impurities, depending on the manufacturing and purification processes.

DMF is stable. It is hygroscopic and easily absorbs water from a humid atmosphere and should therefore be kept under dry nitrogen. High purity DMF, required for acrylic fibres, is best stored in aluminium tanks. DMF does not change under light or oxygen and does not polymerize spontaneously. Temperatures > 350 °C may cause decomposition to form dimethylamine and carbon dioxide, with pressure developing in closed containers (Farhi et al., 1968; US NIOSH, 1978). In a fire involving DMF, or at temperatures > 350 °C, the toxic gases and vapours consist primarily of dimethylamine and carbon monoxide.

Table 1. Physical properties of DMF

Property	Value
Melting point (°C)	- 60.5
Boiling point (°C)	153
Flash point (°C)	58 (closed cup)
	67 (open cup)
Auto-ignition temperature (°C)	445
Density at 25 °C (specific gravity) (g/ml)	0.9445
Relative vapour density	2.51
Vapour pressure (mmHg/kPa)	
at 20 °C	2.65/0.35
at 25 °C	3.7/0.48
at 60 °C	26/3.46
Vapour concentration in saturated air at 25 °C (mg/m^3)	14 800
Explosive limits in air at 20 °C (101 kPa/1 atm./%vol.)	
lower limit	2.2 (70 g/m^3)
upper limit	16 (500 g/m^3)
n-Octanol/water partition coefficient	0.13
Solubility in water	Miscible in all proportions
Solubility in organic solvents	Miscible with ether, ketones, aromatic hydrocarbons, ethanol, but not with aliphatic hydrocarbons
Dielectric constant at 20 °C	36.7

DMF reacts readily with alkylaluminiums. Contact with carbon tetrachloride and other halogenated hydrocarbons, particularly when in contact with iron, as well as contact with strong oxidizing agents (e.g., methylene diisocyanate, halogens, and permanganates) may cause fires and explosions. In acidic solution (pH 3.8), DMF can be nitrosated by sodium nitrate yielding small amounts of N-nitrosodimethylamine (0.04% at 37 °C and 1% at 90 °C).

Identity; properties; analytical methods

2.3 Organoleptic properties

DMF is a colourless liquid with an unpleasant taste and an ammonia-like, specific odour that has poor warning properties (US NIOSH, 1978). The odour threshold for the most sensitive people ranges from 0.12 to 0.15 mg/m^3 (Odoshashvili, 1963; Lazarev & Levina, 1976; Amster et al., 1983; Clay & Spittler, 1983). For some people, the odour threshold has been reported to be as high as 60 mg/m^3 (Leonardous et al., 1965).

2.4 Analytical methods

2.4.1 *Determination of DMF in workplace air*

Colorimetric methods, based on the development of a red colour after the addition of hydroxylamine chloride as alkaline solution, are not specific (Farhi et al., 1968). Lauwerys et al. (1980) described a simple spectrophotometric method for measuring DMF vapour concentrations. Gas-liquid chromatography is now the method of choice (Kimmerle & Eben, 1975a; US NIOSH, 1977; Muravieva & Anvaer, 1979; Brugnone et al., 1980a; Muravieva, 1983; Stransky, 1986). Detector tubes, certified by US NIOSH, or other direct-reading devices calibrated to measure DMF (Krivanek et al., 1978; US NIOSH, 1978) can be used. High-performance liquid chromatographic analysis (Lipski, 1982) can also be used. Mass spectrometric analysis for DMF in expired air has been described by Wilson & Ottley (1981), with a lower limit of detection of 0.5 mg/m^3.

2.4.2 *Determination of DMF and metabolites in biological media*

Barnes & Henry (1974) developed a method for the gas chromatographic determination of NMF (*N*-methylformamide) (thought to be the principal metabolite of DMF) in urine at concentrations of between 5 and 500 µg/litre by either direct injection of the urine or of urine extracts. Methods for simultaneous gas chromatographic determination of DMF and NMF in the same blood sample (0.2 ml) and of DMF, NMF, and formamide in 1 ml 24-h urine have been published by Kimmerle & Eben (1975a) and Muravieva & Anvaer (1979). Similar techniques were reported by

Krivanek et al. (1978), Sanotsky et al. (1978), and Lauwerys et al. (1980), involving primarily the determination of NMF in the urine (Table 2).

2.4.3 Determination of DMF in soil, plants, and food

Analytical methods for the determination of DMF in these media have not been described.

Table 2. Analytical methods for the determination of DMF, NMF (DMF-OH), and formamide (NMF-OH) in urine, blood, and other biological tissues

Biological tissue	Analytical method	Detection limits			Reference
		DMF	NMF (DMF-OH)	Formamide (NMF-OH)	
Urine	gas chromatography		0.5 mg/litre		Barnes & Henry (1974)
	gas chromatography	1.5 mg/litre	1 mg/litre	3.5 mg/litre	Kimmerle & Eben (1975a)
	gas chromatography		0.1 mg/litre		Krivanek et al. (1978)
	gas chromatography	1.5 mg/litre	3 mg/litre	10 mg/litre	Muravieva & Anvaer (1979)
	gas chromatography		0.8 mg/litre		Mráz et al. (1987)
					Lauwerys et al. (1980)
Blood	gas chromatography	1 mg/litre	1.5 mg/litre		Kimmerle & Eben (1975a)
	gas chromatography	0.03 mg/litre	0.3 mg/litre		Sanotsky et al. (1978)
	gas chromatography	1.5 mg/litre	3 mg/litre	10 mg/litre	Muravieva & Anvaer (1979)
	gas chromatography	0.4 mmol/litre			Lundberg et al. (1983)
Liver[a]	gas chromatography	0.2 mmol/kg			Lundberg et al. (1983)
Kidney		0.6 mmol/kg			
Brain		0.3 mmol/kg			
Adrenals		0.9 mmol/kg			

[a] Tissue homogenate.

3. SOURCES OF HUMAN AND ENVIRONMENTAL EXPOSURE

3.1 Natural occurrence

DMF does not occur naturally.

3.2 Man-made sources

3.2.1 Production and uses

3.2.1.1 Production

DMF was first synthesized in 1893 from carbon monoxide and dimethylamine (Kennedy, 1986). It is usually manufactured by a one-stage reaction of carbon monoxide with dimethylamine:

$$CO + (CH_3)_2NH \xrightarrow{\text{catalyst}} (CH_3)_2$$

or by a two-stage reaction with methylformate and dimethylamine (Eberling, 1980):

$$CO + CH_3OH \xrightarrow{\text{catalyst}} HCOOCH_3$$

$$HCOOCH_3 + (CH_3)_2NH \longrightarrow HCON(CH_3)_2 + CH_3OH$$

DMF can also be manufactured from carbon dioxide, hydrogen, and dimethylamine, in the presence of halogen-containing transition metal compounds.

DMF is shipped in tank trucks and tank containers, and is also marketed in 200-kg steel drums. The materials for DMF handling and storage are usually (carbon) steels, austenitic steels, and aluminium. Seals and pipelines should be made of polytetrafluoroethylene, polyethylene, or polypropylene of high relative molecular mass. Ethylene-propylene rubber can also be used.

The world production capacity of DMF is about 225 × 10^3 tonnes/year (Eberling, 1980). Production in the USA in 1979 was 15 000 tonnes. In 1980, NIOSH estimated that 69 000 US workers, in various occupations in 25 major industries, were exposed to DMF.

Data are not available on losses of DMF into the environment and into the ambient air during its production and use.

DMF can be recovered from the air by scrubbing with water and from aqueous solution by distillation.

3.2.1.2 Uses

DMF is a universal industrial solvent, because of its water solubility, organic nature, and high dielectric constant. The main use (65-75%) of DMF is as solvent for acrylic fibres and polyurethanes; 15-20% is used in the production of pharmaceutical products (Eberling, 1980).

DMF is used as:

- a spinning solvent for synthetic textiles, based on polyacrylonitrile or cellulose triacetate;
- a resin, rubber, and polymer solvent;
- a solvent for dyes and pigments for use with textiles, wood, leather, films, paper, and plastics;
- a solvent in pesticide formulations;
- a booster solvent in coating, printing, and adhesive formulations;
- a chemical intermediate, catalyst, and reaction medium in chemical manufacturing and the pharmaceutical industry;
- a solvent in the production of polyurethane and other synthetic leathers, or synthetic rubber;
- a selective absorption and extraction solvent for recovery, purification, absorption, separation, and desulfurization of non-paraffinic compounds from paraffin hydrocarbons;
- in the manufacture of paint stripper components for the removal of vinyl films, epoxy coatings, and varnish finishes; in the production of wire enamels, based on polyamides, polyurethanes, and other polymers;

- in the pigment and dye industry to improve dyeing properties;
- a crystallization solvent in the pharmaceutical industry;
- a solvent for carbonaceous deposit cleaning applications for high-voltage capacitors;
- an oil sludge dispersing agent;
- an anti-stall gasoline additive;
- a laboratory solvent and as a solvent for the extraction of biological material in chemical analysis.

DMF (itself, or as a component in consumer products) is not generally available to the general population (Farhi et al., 1968; Bainova, 1980; Lundberg, 1982; Tanaka & Utsunomiya, 1982; Barral-Chamaillard & Rouzioux, 1983; Kennedy, 1986; US EPA, 1986).

Because of its hepatotoxicity, DMF is not used as a solvent in pharmaceutical or cosmetic products.

DMF has been approved by the US FDA as a component of adhesives, for use in the packaging, transport, or storage of food.

DMF is present in some registered pesticides as an inert solvent.

4. ENVIRONMENTAL TRANSPORT, DISTRIBUTION, AND TRANSFORMATION

4.1 Transport and distribution between media

4.1.1 Air

DMF is stable in air. Concentrations in ambient air are related to its industrial use. No data have been found on the rates of reaction of DMF with hydroxyl radicals, ozone, or other atmospheric pollutants. Darnall et al. (1976) reported DMF to have a half-life of 9.9 days in a polluted atmosphere. In oxidizing smog-chamber studies (Laity et al., 1973; Farley, 1977; Sickles et al., 1980), no photochemical oxidation of DMF occurred. The ultraviolet (UV) absorption spectrum for DMF indicated no absorption > 290 nm (Grasselli, 1973), showing that no photodegradation should be expected in the environment. The water solubility of DMF suggests that it should be easily removed from air by rainfall.

The DMF levels in the air of working environments depend on the rate of usage, technology, and industrial hygiene practices (Aldyreva & Gafurov, 1980; Brugnone et al., 1980a; Lauwerys et al., 1980; Yonemoto & Suzuki, 1980; Koudela & Spazier, 1981; Taccola et al., 1981; Paoletti & Iannaccone, 1982; Tomasini et al., 1983; Sala et al., 1984; Kennedy, 1986; US EPA, 1986).

4.1.2 Water

According to Eberling (1980), aqueous solutions of DMF undergo slight hydrolysis at neutral pH. After 120 h of refluxing, only 0.17% of a 50% solution was hydrolysed. The hydrolysis of DMF is accelerated by acids and alkalis. No data about the oxidation or photodegradation of DMF are available.

DMF is susceptible to biodegradation by activated sludges, though an acclimation period is usually required. Water from the Vistula River was reported to biodegrade DMF, as was an unspecified bacterial culture isolated from soil exposed to petroleum + petroleum products (Chromek et al., 1983). Dojlido (1979) reported that, in an activated sludge system, 100% of the 70 mg DMF/litre was degraded in 38 days. In a river die-away test, under light aeration conditions,

28 mg DMF/litre were degraded in the water with a lag time of 2 days. The lag time decreased when acclimatized microorganisms were used in the test.

Chromek et al. (1983) determined the changes in respiration rate in algal cultures of *Scenedesmus quadricauda*, after treatment with 1000 mg DMF/litre. DMF degradation via dimethylamine to ammonia occurred within 3 days. The rate of DMF degradation to ammonia depended on the degree of adaptation of the heterotrophic mixed cultures (activated sludge) and varied between 35 and 70 mg/g per h. The dimethylamine decomposition rate was about 25 mg/g per h.

Gubser (1969) reported that, in a continuous-flow activated sludge system, DMF was reduced by 90-100% within 10 days at concentrations of 20 and 50 mg/litre, and within 28 days at a concentration of 81 mg/litre. Chromek et al. (1983) found that the alga *Scenedesmus quadricauda* in cultures was able to degrade DMF to dimethylamine and ammonia in 3 days. The DMF concentration tested was about 1000 mg/litre; this corresponds to values seen in industrial effluents. After the formation of an adaptive enzymatic system, the DMF concentration decreased at a constant rate of about 40 mg/g per h. Adaptation of the culture resulted in an enhanced rate of degradation. *Pseudomonas* sp., *Pseudomonas* sp.II, and *Vibrio aeromonas*, isolated from sewage effluents, degraded DMF (US EPA, 1986). Begert (1975) proposed several series of aerobic bacterial systems, which eliminated more than 90% of the DMF in the sewage from a chemical textile plant.

The complete water solubility and low *n*-octanol/water partition coefficient (Table 1) of DMF suggest that adsorption on sediments in water is not an important environmental process. DMF is not expected to evaporate from the aquatic environment to any significant rate because of its volatility and high water solubility (US EPA, 1986).

4.1.3 Soil

Contamination of soil with DMF may occur through spillage or leakage during its production, transport, storage, or use. DMF's high solubility in water and its low *n*-octanol/water partition coefficient show that it can seep down into soil and potentially into ground water. DMF was completely biodegraded by a bacterial culture, isolated from soil that had been in contact with low levels of petroleum and petroleum products for several years. This culture was used for the purification of waste waters containing 250 mg DMF/litre in an aerated tank; the addition of activated sludge for 18 h resulted in the biodegradation of 94% of the DMF (Romadina, 1975).

4.1.4 Bioaccumulation

Sasaki (1978) found that DMF did not bioaccumulate in the carp; the low partition coefficient was considered to be the explanation.

5. ENVIRONMENTAL LEVELS AND HUMAN EXPOSURE

5.1 Environmental levels

5.1.1 Air

Air-monitoring for DMF was conducted at distances ranging from 25 to 300 m from an artificial fibre plant in the USSR. Odoshashvili (1963) found that DMF levels were only below the proposed allowable limit of 0.03 mg/m^3 at 300 m from the plant.

Residents of private homes within a 0.5 mile radius of a chemical waste recycling site complained of unpleasant odours. DMF was found to be the major atmospheric contaminant in concentrations of up to 0.12 mg/m^3, but it originated primarily from the industrial sites nearby and not from the soil or the waste site (Clay & Spittler, 1983). Amster et al. (1983) studied another abandoned chemical waste facility in the USA, in response to complaints from nearby residents about odour, with similar results, i.e., air levels of 0.024-0.15 mg DMF/m^3 originated from a neighbouring industry.

5.1.2 Water

Very low concentrations of DMF were found in effluent waters from sewage-treatment plants or municipal sewage-treatment systems (US EPA, 1986). A concentration of 2 µg/litre was measured in a sample taken from a sewage-treatment plant on the western shore of Lake Michigan. Ewing et al. (1977) examined 204 water samples from 14 heavily industrialized river basins in the USA. DMF was found in only one sample, at a concentration of 2 µg/litre. Samples of 63 effluent and 22 intake waters from various chemical manufacturers were collected in areas throughout the USA (Perry et al., 1979) and analysed for organic pollutants. Over 570 compounds were tentatively identified, of which 33 were important pollutants. DMF was detected once at a concentration < 10 µg/litre.

Chromek et al. (1983) reported that DMF concentrations of approximately 1000 mg/litre were found in effluents from the production of synthetic leather.

5.1.3 Soil

No data are available on DMF levels in soil and plants.

5.2 General population exposure

No data are available on exposure of the general population to DMF.

However, DMF may be a component of coatings, adhesives, engine degreasing agents, and photographic developers for consumer use.

Exposure through the use of DMF in food processing, food packaging, and pesticides may occur, but data are not available.

5.3 Occupational exposure

5.3.1 Concentrations in the workplace air

DMF is not highly volatile and is manufactured in closed systems. Data on DMF concentrations in plants manufacturing DMF are not available.

Concentrations of DMF in the workplace air in various industrial applications are listed in Table 3. In most cases, the mean concentrations are less than 30 mg/m^3, but certain jobs, particularly those involving mixing operations, result in higher concentrations. The cleaning of equipment or tanks that have contained DMF can involve exposure to levels of up to 147 mg/m^3. Kang-de & Hui-lan (1981) reported an unusually high DMF concentration of 4525 mg/m^3 during repairs following an accident. The ranges of concentration reported vary considerably, but the time of sampling is not generally specified. The highest values have been found during repair or maintenance work, in accidents, and where batch sampling (opening the reactor system) was being conducted.

Table 3. DMF concentrations in air in various industrial applications

Factory product	Job description	Mean DMF concentrations (mg/m³)	Range of DMF concentrations (mg/m³)	Reference
Polyacrylic fibres	spinning line - maintenance	-	1-46.6	Lauwerys et al. (1980)
Artificial leather	various (pre-improvement)	-	0-60	Aldyreva & Gafurov (1980)
	various (post-improvement)		1/3 samples below detection	
	production	5.3	1.9-8.3	Brugnone et al. (1980a)
	production (highest in mixing)	> 30	< 150	Taccola et al. (1981)
	production - normal	4.2-66		Paoletti & Iannaccone (1982)
	opening reactor	-	< 549	
	maintenance of rollers	-	< 120	
	production - mixing	> 34		Tomasini et al. (1983)
	soaking and drying	12.1 (± 40.2)		Bortsevich (1984)
	coating and colouring	32.3 (± 98.7)		
	mixing resins	22.7 and 85.2	2-117	Sala et al. (1984)
	spreading "transfer" system	33.8	8-72	
	spreading "coagulate" system	14	2-49	
	tank cleaning	86.3	9-147	
	machine cleaning	24.1	12-35	
Surface-treating agents	handlers	0-15.4	-	Yonemoto & Suzuki (1980)
Solvents	-	often > 30	peak 105-600	Lyle et al. (1979)
Synthetic rubber	repairing, accidents, sampling with system opened,	-	9.5-4525	Kang-de & Hui-lan (1981)
	extracting	< 10	-	
Unspecified chemicals	unspecified	-	50-250	Koudela & Spazier (1981)

Environmental levels and human exposure

5.3.2 Dermal exposure

The relative importance of dermal exposure to liquid or vapour DMF (versus inhalation of vapour) was studied by Aldyreva & Gafurov (1980), Lauwerys et al. (1980), Bortsevich (1984), and Sala et al. (1984).

Lauwerys et al. (1980) studied 7 workers from a spinning mill in a polyacrylic fibre factory. During the first week, the workers wore gloves and during the second week, a barrier cream was applied twice each day to the hands and forearms. On the first day of the third week, the skin was not protected, but the workers were equipped with self-contained breathing equipment. The average *N*-methylformamide (NMF) concentration in the urine at the end of the day, when there was no dermal protection, was about 3 times higher than that during the first week. Eight hours after the start of exposure without skin protection, one worker reported abdominal pains; a second worker had to stop working 48 h later because of severe gastric pain. Hence, from the second day, the workers were requested to resume wearing their impermeable gloves. Urinary NMF concentrations returned to the values found during the first week. This convinced the workers of the need to avoid all contact with the DMF solution and to use protective gloves correctly. The study also showed that gloves were more effective than silicone or glycerol barrier creams in preventing skin absorption of DMF.

In a new plant producing artificial leather, Aldyreva et al. (1980) found DMF in nearly all washings from the operators' hands.

According to Bortsevich (1984), the quantity of DMF absorbed through the skin might be twice the quantity taken up through inhalation. The author reported significant DMF concentrations in the skin washings from the palms of hands, shoulders, back, thighs, and abdomen. Part of the dermal uptake of DMF may result from its presence in the air and part from contaminated clothing.

Sala et al. (1984) reported that the total daily excretion of NMF (DMF-OH[a] and NMF) in the 24-h urine samples of a worker who

---

[a] DMF-OH = *N*-hydroxymethyl-*N*-methylformamide.

usually cleaned the tanks in a factory where artificial polyurethane leathers were produced, was 95-725 mg or 35-390 mg NMF/litre. This is higher than would have been expected in a subject with a mean airborne exposure of 100 mg DMF/m^3. The worker usually operated without using any personal protection.

Penetration through various glove materials has been studied. Breakthrough time was > 480 min for butyl rubber, 6-66 min for neoprene, and 5-22 min for polyvinylchloride and polyvinyl alcohol (Henry & Schlatter, 1981).

Similarly, Sansone & Tewari (1978) showed that < 0.1% DMF passed through neoprene gloves, 0.1-1% through natural rubber gloves, 1-10% through nitrile gloves, and > 10% through polyvinylchloride gloves, in half an hour.

6. KINETICS AND METABOLISM

6.1 Animal studies

6.1.1 Absorption

Sanotsky et al. (1978) determined DMF concentrations in the blood of rats, 24 h after the oral administration of 200-4000 mg DMF/kg body weight and found mean blood levels ranging from 40 to 1870 mg/litre. DMF is readily absorbed via inhalation and dermally. Maximal blood and tissue concentrations were observed in rats up to 3 h after exposure to 438 and 6015 mg DMF/m^3 (Kimmerle & Eben, 1975a) or to 1690 and 6700 mg DMF/m^3 (Lundberg et al., 1983). According to Massmann (1956), at least 0.8 ml of 100% DMF was absorbed through 14 cm^2 of exposed skin of the tails of rats in the course of 8 h, which is equivalent to an absorption rate of about 57 mg/cm^2 per 8 h.

6.1.2 Distribution

Twenty-four hours after an ip dose of ^{14}C-DMF in male rats, about 4% of the radioactivity was recovered in the blood, less than 1% in the brain, heart, lungs, stomach, intestines, spleen, and kidneys, and 1-3% in the liver, adipose tissue, and muscles (Scailteur & Lauwerys, 1984).

Kimmerle & Eben (1975a) studied DMF and NMF (DMF-OH)[a] concentrations in the blood of rats and dogs after single and repeated respiratory exposure. At the highest airborne concentration (6015 mg/m^3), DMF was still detectable in the blood of male rats up to 2 days after the end of a 3-h exposure. At lower concentrations, DMF levels in the blood decreased rapidly (Table 4). After 3-h exposure to 63 mg/m^3 or 6-h exposure to 87 mg/m^3, similar levels of NMF were found in the blood at the end of the periods of exposure,

---

[a] DMF = dimethylformamide;
DMF-OH = N-hydroxymethyl-N-methylformamide;
NMF = N-methylformamide;
NMF-OH = N-hydroxymethylformamide;
F = formamide.

but no NMF was detectable 3 h after the end of exposure. Only after a 3-h exposure to a very high concentration (6015 mg/m^3) did NMF levels in blood continue to increase for the 2 days following exposure (Table 4).

Table 4. Concentrations of DMF and NMF in the blood of male rats after a single inhalation exposure

Hours after end of exposure	Inhalation exposure to DMF (3 h)					
	6015 mg/m^3		438 mg/m^3		63 mg/m^3	
	DMF	NMF	DMF	NMF	DMF	NMF
	(mg/litre)		(mg/litre)		(mg/litre)	
0	1190	11.5	25.7	7.3	ND^a	2.5
0.5	1166	12.1	21.7	6.9		1.9
1	1329	15.8	20.7	10.2		1.2
2.5	1275	20.9	10.5	11.8		0.5
4.5	1322	25.9	1.8	10.6		ND
21	824	50.3				
45	46	84.3				

^{a} ND = not detectable.

Blood concentrations of DMF in male dogs also decreased rapidly following a 6-h single exposure. However, NMF could be detected in the blood at higher concentrations and for a longer period of time after exposure (Table 5).

When male rats were exposed to 1050 ± 126 mg/m^3, 6 h/day, for 5 days, the levels of DMF and NMF in the blood returned to ND levels before each consecutive exposure. However, when male dogs were exposed to 177 ± 36 mg NFM/m^3, 6 h/day, for 5 days, NMF accumulated in the blood (10 mg/litre, 2 h after the first exposure; 30 mg/litre, 3 h after the fifth exposure). In contrast, in female dogs, exposed to 69 ± 12 mg/m^3, 6 h/day, for 5 days, the daily NMF concentration in the blood remained almost constant, returning to a low level of about 1-1.5 mg/ml, before each new exposure.

Finally, in male and female dogs exposed to 63 ± 9 mg/m^3, 6 h/day, for 5 days a week over 4 weeks, DMF levels went back to ND before each new exposure. There was no accumulation of NMF.

Table 5. Concentrations of DMF and NMF in the blood of male dogs after a single inhalation exposure

Hours after end of exposure	Inhalation exposure to DMF (6 h)			
	513 ± 114 mg/m^3		60 ± 9 mg/m^3	
	DMF (mg/litre)	NMF (mg/litre)	DMF (mg/litre)	NMF (mg/litre)
0	51.6	9.7	7.4	10.5
0.5	54.9	13.7	5.6	11.9
1	47.7	14.9	4.1	12.1
2	39.4	17.4	0.7	13.3
3	38.7	23.6	ND[a]	13.3
27				3.1

[a] ND = not detectable.

The weekly average concentrations of NMF were slightly higher in males than in females.

Lundberg et al. (1983) measured DMF and NMF concentrations in various organs of the rat after a single 4-h inhalation exposure to 1690 or 6700 DMF mg/m^3; DMF and NMF were distributed uniformly throughout the tissues (Tables 6 and 7). Blood levels of NMF (DMF-OH) for the first 3 h following exposure were lower after exposure to 6700 mg/m^3 than after exposure to 1690 mg/m^3 (Table 6 and 7). The authors suggested that high DMF doses inhibit DMF biotransformation. This interpretation is supported by the results of Kimmerle & Eben (1975a), who reported that NMF concentrations in the blood (11-21 mg/litre) during the first 3 h following a 3-h exposure to 6015 mg DMF/m^3 were lower than those following a 6-h exposure to 513 mg/m^3.

6.1.3 Metabolic transformation

After iv injection of DMF in cats, Massman (1956) found that only a small amount of the compound was excreted unchanged in the urine. He could not detect any hydrolysis of the amide to dimethylamine and formic acid. Barnes & Ranta (1972) identified a urinary metabolite, NMF, in the urine of rats treated with sc injections of DMF.

Table 6. Concentrations of DMF and NMF in rat tissues after a 4-h exposure to 6700 mg DMF/m³

Hours after end of exposure	Blood (mg/litre)		Liver		Kidney (mmol/kg)		Brain		Adrenals	
	DMF	NMF	DMF	NMF	DMF	NMF	DMF	NMF	DMF	NMF
0	965	< 24	9.8	< 0.3	11.0	0.8	11.4	0.4	8.6	< 1.0
3	1089	< 24	11.7	0.5	12.8	< 0.6	2.7	< 0.3	8.8	< 1.0
6	950	71	10.1	0.7	11.5	1.3	10.1	0.5	9.0	1.2
20	263	295	2.6	1.9	3.1	2.3	1.5	2.1	1.9	1.9
48	< 29	< 24	< 0.2	< 0.3	< 0.6	< 0.6	< 0.3	< 0.3	< 0.9	< 1.0

Table 7. Concentrations of DMF and NMF in rat tissues after a 4-h exposure to 1690 mg DMF/m³

Hours after end of exposure	Blood (mg/litre)		Liver		Kidney (mmol/kg)		Brain		Adrenals	
	DMF	NMF	DMF	NMF	DMF	NMF	DMF	NMF	DMF	NMF
0	373	41	2.8	0.5	3.1	0.9	3.1	0.5	2.1	< 1.0
3	205	47	1.8	0.5	2.8	0.9	2.0	0.6	1.6	< 1.0
6	197	47	1.8	0.6	2.0	1.2	1.9	0.7	1.5	1.0
20	< 29	< 24	< 0.5	< 0.3	< 0.6	0.6	< 0.3	< 0.3	< 0.9	< 1.0
48	< 29	< 24	< 0.5	< 0.3	< 0.6	0.6	< 0.3	< 0.3	< 0.9	< 1.0

After single or repeated respiratory exposure to DMF, Kimmerle & Eben (1975a) identified NMF and formamide in the urine of rats and dogs. The authors proposed a model of successive N-demethylations of DMF.

In *in vitro* studies, Barnes & Ranta (1972) measured a low level of formaldehyde, when rat liver homogenates were incubated with DMF in the presence of an NADPH-generating system. They concluded that DMF was N-demethylated in the liver with the help of microsomal enzymes. This was in agreement with previous *in vivo* findings.

Later on, however, it was shown that the incubation of various rat tissues with DMF did not release formaldehyde *in vitro*. Furthermore, neither formaldehyde nor any other monocarbon derivative (CO, CH_3OH, CH_4, $HCOOH$) was detected, when DMF was incubated with fortified liver microsomes. However, a metabolite determined by gas chromatography (GC) was identified as NMF. This led to speculation that DMF-OH was a probable metabolite of DMF that was broken down (demethylated) to form NMF during gas chromatographic analysis (Scailteur et al., 1984).

Brindley et al. (1983) indicated that a stable precursor of formaldehyde was present in the urine of mice treated with DMF.

Direct evidence that DMF-OH is a metabolite of DMF was only obtained by investigating urine samples of animals treated with DMF. DMF-OH was identified in rat urine using HPLC combined with chemical ionization mass spectrometry (Scailteur et al., 1984) and in mouse urine high-field H-NMR spectroscopy and radio thin layer chromatography (Kestell et al., 1986).

Using GC combined with mass spectrometry, Scailteur & Lauwerys (1984a,b) showed that besides the major metabolite, DMF-OH, a small amount of NMF could also be identified in the urine of DMF-treated rats. This was confirmed by Kestell et al. (1986) using H-NMR spectroscopy. Thus when urine samples are analysed after DMF administration, using gas chromatography, the combination of DMF-OH + NMF is determined as NMF and the combination of hydroxymethylformamide (NMF-OH) + formamide, as formamide (Scailteur et al., 1984). Using GC/MS, Scailteur & Lauwerys (1984a,b) could not identify NMF in the urine of

DMF-OH-treated rats. The authors therefore suggested that NMF is not a product of DMF-OH biotransformation, but is directly formed from DMF.

Hepatectomy markedly reduced the *in vivo* transformation of DMF into DMF-OH, confirming that the liver is the main site of metabolic degradation (Scailteur et al., 1984).

In parallel with the hypothesis of Lundberg et al. (1983) that high doses of DMF could inhibit its biotransformation, Scailteur et al. (1984) showed that the urinary excretion of metabolites (DMF-OH + NMF, NMF-OH + F) was the same, following 2 daily ip injections of 0.5 mg/kg body weight or 2 daily ip injections of 1 ml/kg.

Scailteur & Lauwerys (1984a) studied the mechanism of the *in vitro* and *in vivo* oxidative biotransformation of DMF. Addition of catalase or superoxide dismutase to liver microsomes, incubated with DMF, decreased the level of DMF-OH production. *In vitro* and *in vivo*, DMF transformation was also diminished in the presence of radical scavengers, such as dimethylsulfoxide, tert-butyl alcohol, hydroquinone, and trichloroacetonitrile. Addition of IRON/EDTA[a] to microsomes, incubated with DMF *in vitro*, stimulated DMF oxidation. The authors concluded that the metabolic transformation of DMF to DMF-OH involved hydroxyl radicals.

Metabolites, other than DMF-OH (NMF) and NMF-OH (F), appear to be formed from DMF. Indeed, about 20% of an ip dose was recovered in the urine of mice (Brindley et al., 1983) and rats (Scailteur & Lauwerys, 1984a,b), as unidentified chemicals.

Kestell et al. (1986, 1987) identified low levels of methylamine and dimethylamine in the urine of DMF-treated mice (about 4%).

A metabolic transformation scheme is presented in Fig. 1, based on the above data.

---

[a] EDTA = ethylene diamine tetra acetate.

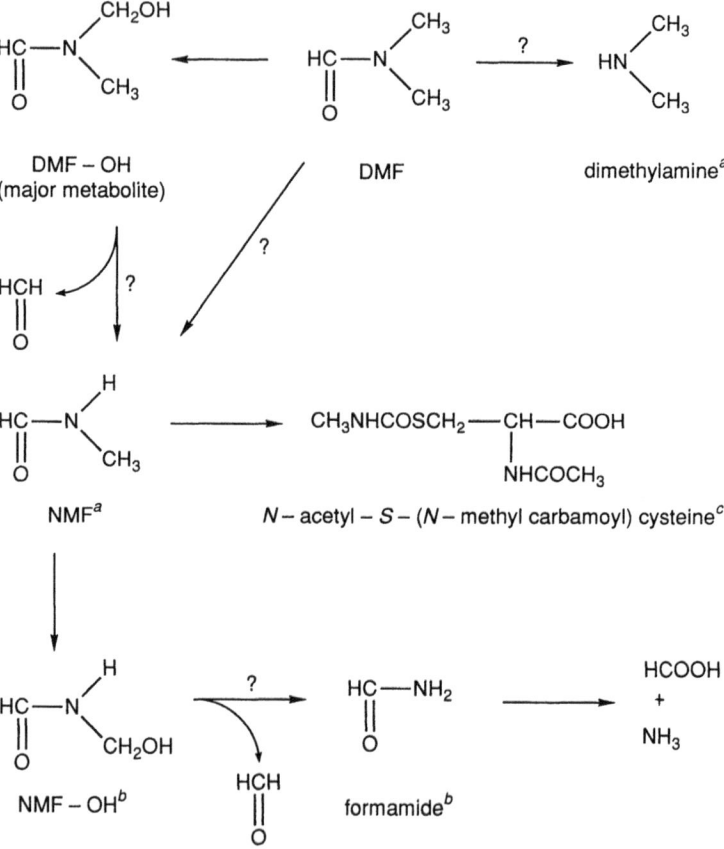

Fig. 1. DMF biotransformations

[a] unequivocally identified in urine of treated animals
[b] identified in urine as NMF – OH or NMF – OH + formamide
[c] identified in urine of animals treated with NMF

Adapted from Scailteur (1984).

6.1.4 Elimination and excretion

The transformation and excretion of DMF in rodents is rapid. When ^{14}C-labelled DMF in 0.1 ml saline was injected ip at 6.8 mmol/kg body weight in mice, about 83% of the radioactivity was recovered in the urine within 24 h following injection. Of this amount, only 5% was unchanged DMF and 56% was C-hydroxylated or N-demethylated derivatives. About 18% of the dose was excreted in the form of unknown chemicals (Brindley et al., 1983).

Similarly, 24 h after ip injection of 400 mg DMF/kg body weight in 0.2 ml saline in mice, about 56% of the dose was excreted in the urine as DMF-OH and only 5% as unchanged DMF (Kestell et al., 1986).

Within 72 h of an ip administration of 1 ml ^{14}C-DMF/kg to male or female rats, 70% of the injected radioactivity was recovered in the urine. Approximately 15% was excreted as unchanged DMF, 50% as DMF-OH (NMF), and 5% as NMF-OH (F). About 20% was excreted as unidentified metabolite(s) (Scailteur & Lauwerys, 1984a,b).

After oral exposure to DMF (40-2000 mg/kg), Sanotsky et al. (1978) determined that about 6% of the dose was excreted in 24 h.

The elimination of DMF, NMF (DMF-OH), and formamide (NMF-OH) was measured after single or repeated inhalation exposure in rats and dogs (Kimmerle & Eben, 1975a). Twenty-four hours after a single exposure to 63 mg NMF/m^3 for 3 h, or 87 mg/m^3 for 6 h, no NMF was found in the urine of male rats. Under the same conditions, exposure to 513 mg/m^3 for 6 h or to 6015 mg/m^3 for 3 h led to excretion of 4 mg and 14 mg NMF (DMF-OH), respectively, during the 24 h following the start of exposure. Only in the last case was DMF also measured in the urine. After repeated exposure of male rats to DMF (1050 mg/m^3, 6 h/day, for 5 days), urinary levels of NMF (DMF-OH) remained practically constant for the first 3 days, then slightly decreased from the fourth day of exposure. Excretion of F (NMF-OH) was much lower than excretion of NMF (DMF-OH).

While no accumulation of urinary NMF (DMF-OH) was observed in male rats, male dogs exposed to 177 mg DMF/m^3 (6 h/day for 5 days) excreted increasing concentrations of NMF (DMF-OH) (36 mg/24 h after the first inhalation; 87 mg/24 h after the 4th inhalation). Urinary excretion of formamide (NMF-OH) varied between 10 and 20 mg/24 h. Excretion of unchanged DMF was very low (< 2 mg/24 h). However, in female dogs exposed to 69 mg/m^3 (6 h/day for 5 days), no urinary accumulation of NMF or F was observed. When male or female rats were exposed for 4 weeks to 63 mg/m^3 (6 h/day, 5 days per week), NMF and F concentrations in the urine remained practically constant during the exposure period. Male dogs generally excreted slightly higher levels of metabolites than female dogs (Kimmerle & Eben, 1975a).

In rats treated with repeated, high, ip doses of DMF (4 daily injections of 1 ml/kg body weight), Scailteur et al. (1984) showed that females excreted higher amounts of unchanged DMF than males. The pattern of metabolite (NMF, F) excretion was similar in both sexes after single or repeated ip administration.

6.1.5 Metabolic interaction between DMF and ethanol

DMF and ethanol appear to interact metabolically.

The alterations in blood metabolites depend on the dose of DMF, the time interval between DMF and ethanol administration, and the respective routes of administration.

The various studies performed are summarized in Table 8. Blood concentrations of DMF and NMF, ethanol, and acetaldehyde were measured using GC methods.

The influence of DMF on ethanol oxidation might be explained, at least partially, by its inhibitory effect on the activity of alcohol dehydrogenase *in vitro* and *in vivo* (Sharkawi, 1979) and aldehyde dehydrogenase *in vivo* (Elovaara et al., 1983).

Table 8. Metabolic interaction between DMF and ethanol

Species	Ethanol dose (route)	Time of administration	DMF dose (route)	Effects on blood concentrations of: DMF and NMF	Effects on blood concentrations of: Ethanol and acetaldehyde	Reference
Rat	0.2 g/kg (oral)	immediately before DMF exposure	312 mg/m³ 2 h (inhalation)	No effects on DMF and NMF	not measured	Eben & Kimmerle (1976)
Rat	2 g/kg (oral)	immediately before DMF exposure	261 or 627 mg/m³ 2 h (inhalation)	DMF increased NMF formation	not measured	Eben & Kimmerle (1976)
Rat	2 g/kg per day for 5 days (oral)	daily immediately before DMF exposure	about 600 mg/m³ 2 h/day 5 days (inhalation)	DMF increased NMF formation	ethanol increased	Eben & Kimmerle (1976)
Dog	2 g/kg (oral)	immediately before DMF exposure	about 630 mg/m³ 2 h (inhalation)	DMF increased NMF decreased	not measured	Eben & Kimmerle (1976)
Dog	2 g/kg (oral)	immediately after DMF exposure	630 mg/m³ 2 h (inhalation)	DMF increased NMF decreased	not measured	Eben & Kimmerle (1976)
Rat	2 g/kg (oral)	1 h after last DMF exposure	3000 mg/m³ 4 h/day 3 days (inhalation)	not measured	acetaldehyde increased	Hanasono et al. (1977)
Rat	2 g/kg (oral)	1 h after last DMF exposure	6000 mg/m³ 4 h/day 3 days (inhalation)	not measured	ethanol increased acetaldehyde decreased	Hanasono et al. (1977)

Table 8. (continued)

Species	Ethanol dose (route)	Time of administration	DMF dose (route)	Effects on blood concentrations of: DMF and NMF	Effects on blood concentrations of: Ethanol and acetaldehyde	Reference
Mouse	1 g/kg (ip)	2 h after DMF exposure	1.2 ml/kg (ip)	not measured	ethanol increased	Sharkawi (1980)
Rat	2 g/kg (oral)	3 h after DMF exposure	0.15 g/kg (oral)	not measured	ethanol increased acetaldehyde decreased	Hanasono et al. (1977)
Rat	2 g/kg (oral)	18 h after DMF exposure	0.15 g/kg (oral)	not measured	acetaldehyde* increased	Hanasono et al. (1977)
Rat	2 g/kg (oral)	18 h after DMF exposure	1.5 g/kg (oral)	not measured	ethanol increased	Hanasono et al. (1977)
Rat	2 g/kg (oral)	24 h after last DMF exposure	3000 mg/m^3 4 h/day 3 days (inhalation)	not measured	acetaldehyde increased	Hanasono et al. (1977)
Rat	2 g/kg (oral)	24 h after last DMF exposure	12 000 mg/m^3 4 h/day 3 days (inhalation)	not measured	acetaldehyde increased	Hanasono et al. (1977)

* Increased acetaldehyde level observed after this dose of DMF was equivalent to that produced by an equimolar dose of disulfiram (antabuse).

6.2 Human studies

6.2.1 Absorption, distribution, metabolism, excretion

In vitro studies on excised human skin (Bortsevich, 1984) showed a relationship between the amount of DMF absorbed through the dermal barrier and the DMF concentrations in water, as well as the exposure time. DMF enhances its own penetration. Some of the results are given in Table 9. They are of practical value, because such solutions are used in synthetic fibre production.

After respiratory exposure to DMF, lung retention in workers in an artificial leather factory was 72% (Brugnone, 1980a,b).

Table 9. Quantities of DMF absorbed in *in vitro* studies on excised human skin

Exposure period (h)	DMF solutions in water			
	100%	60%	30%	15%
	% DMF absorbed through the skin (mg/cm^2)			
0.5	0.046	ND^a	ND^a	ND^a
1-1.5	7.400	0.035	0.013	0.006
2-2.5	20.550	0.087	0.048	0.009
3-3.5	40.810	0.222	0.097	0.017
4-4.5	51.730	0.300	0.160	0.069

^{a} ND = Not detectable.

The relative importance of skin versus inhalation for DMF absorption was studied in volunteers by Maxfield et al. (1975), Kimmerle & Eben (1975a), and Krivanek et al. (1978) (section 6.2.3.1).

As in animals, the major human metabolite of DMF has been reported to be DMF-OH and not NMF. However, it is measured as NMF when using gas chromatography including the small amount of NMF excreted in the urine (Scailteur & Lauwerys, 1987).

Kinetics and metabolism

When a male volunteer inhaled the DMF vapours that were produced over liquid DMF in a beaker for 6 h, Mraz & Turecek (1987) identified the metabolite N-acetyl-S-(N-methylcarbamoyl) cysteine in the urine.

Malonova & Bardodej (1983) reported a possible increase in the urinary excretion of mercapturates in workers exposed to unknown concentrations of DMF (approximately twice the excretion in controls (smokers)).

6.2.2 *The influence of ethanol on DMF metabolism in human volunteers*

Eben & Kimmerle (1976) exposed 4 subjects via inhalation to DMF (159 mg/m^3) for 2 h with, and without, ingestion of 19 g ethanol (50 ml 38% gin), 10 min before they inhaled the DMF. No changes in DMF concentrations in blood were found. The comparatively lower NMF concentrations in the blood of subjects with combined exposure to ethanol and DMF indicated that the ethanol decreased the biotransformation of DMF. No significant differences in the blood levels of ethanol and acetaldehyde were detected in subjects with, or without, ethanol exposure, which differed from the effects observed in animal studies. The authors suggested that this was because of the relatively low concentrations of DMF used in the human studies.

6.2.3 *Biological monitoring of workers*

N-Hydroxymethyl-N-methylformamide (DMF-OH) has been identified as the main urinary metabolite of DMF. It is measured, using gas chromatography, as NMF together with the small proportion of NMF excreted in the urine. Some results of studies on the correlation between exposure levels to DMF and NMF excretion in workers and human volunteers are given in Table 10.

6.2.3.1 *Determination of NMF in the urine*

NMF (DMF-OH) in the urine is a sensitive biological parameter of human DMF exposure. NMF levels in the urine are usually greater at the end of the shift than on the morning after the exposure.

Table 10. NMF levels in urine as a test for DMF exposure

Subjects	DMF concentrations in the air	NMF concentrations in the urine	Time of sampling	Reference
4 volunteers	78 ± 24 mg/m³ [a] 261 ± 75 mg/m³ [a] 63 ± 12 mg/m³ [b]	24 mg/24 h 97.4 mg/24 h 30 mg/24 h		Kimmerle & Eben (1975a)
4 volunteers	159 ± 96 mg/m³ [a]	44.8 mg/24 h		Eben & Kimmerle (1976)
4 volunteers	32.4 ± 2.1 mg/m³ [a,c]	5 mg/24 h		Maxfield et al. (1975)
8 volunteers	26.4 ± 0.9 mg/m³ [b]	2.5 mg/24 h		Krivanek et al. (1978)
22 workers	13 mg/m³ [b]	20-40 mg/g creatinine	post-shift samples	Lauwerys et al. (1980)
9 workers	15.4 mg/m³ [b]	0.4-19.6 mg/24 h		Yonemoto & Suzuki (1980)
85 workers	30-150 mg/m³ [b,c]	0.104-0.224 mg/ml		Aldyreva et al. (1980)
23 workers	above 30 mg/m³ [b]	20-40 mg/24 h		Taccola et al. (1981)
2 volunteers	30 mg/m³ [b]	102.6 µmol/8 h		Wicarova & Dadak (1981)
39 workers		217.5 µmol/24 h		
30 workers	14-86.3 mg/m³ [b]	12-188.3 mg/g creatinine	4 h after the work shift different work areas	Sala et al. (1984)

[a] Single inhalation exposure to DMF (2, 4, or 6 h/day).
[b] Repeated inhalation exposure to DMF (6, 7, 7.5 h/day).
[c] Dermal absorption.

Lauwerys et al. (1980) compared a group of 22 male workers from the spinning mill in a polyacrylic fibre plant with 28 controls. The workers in the spinning department wore gloves and long sleeves, but did not have any respiratory protection. Spot urine samples were collected before, and after, the work shift for 5 consecutive days, to determine NMF and creatinine concentrations. NMF was not detected in the urine of control workers, who were not exposed to DMF. There was a poor correlation, on an individual basis, between the integrated DMF exposure and the NMF concentration in the urine collected at the end of the shift, or in that collected before resuming work the following day. However, on a group basis, there was a good correlation between the intensity of exposure and NMF levels in the urine collected at the end of the shift.

In a second study in the polyacrylic fibre plant, Lauwerys et al. (1980) studied the NMF levels in the urine of 7 workers for 3 weeks, when different types of personal protective devices were used. Absorption of DMF vapours through the skin was more important than through inhalation. In the absence of skin contact, a concentration of 40-50 mg NMF/g creatinine, in post-shift samples, corresponded to an average concentration of DMF vapour of 13 mg/m^3 (45 ppm) during a 6-h exposure period.

Yonemoto & Suzuki (1980) studied the relationship between the individual occupational exposure to DMF and the amount of NMF in the urine of 9 male workers who handled polyurethane surface-treating agents for synthetic leather. The time-weighted average individual exposures ranged from 0 to 15.4 mg DMF/m^3. The amount of NMF excreted daily ranged from 0.4 to 19.56 mg/24 h. The excretion rate of NMF (mg/h) increased from the beginning of exposure and reached a maximum in the urine samples collected in the evening. The relationship between the total daily NMF excretion in the urine and the level of exposure was represented as a linear regression, indicating that the best biological index of DMF exposure is the determination of NMF in the 24-h urine (Fig. 2). At an 8-h integrated DMF exposure of 15 mg/m^3, the NMF level in the urine of the workers was less than 20 mg/24 h. This value is higher than those obtained for volunteers (Kimmerle & Eben, 1975b; Krivanek et al., 1978) or for workers (Lauwerys et al., 1980). Yonemoto & Suzuki (1980) stated that the difference might be due to dermal absorption of DMF, because the workers did not use protective gloves or special working overalls.

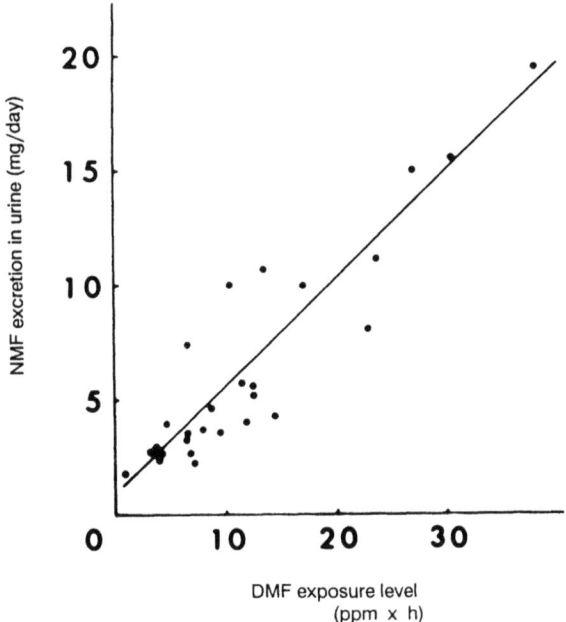

Fig. 2. The relationship between the corrected level of individual exposure to DMF and the total amount of NMF excreted in urine.
From: Yonemoto & Suzuki (1980).

Wicarova & Dadak (1981) studied the relationship between the amount of NMF in the shift urine (8 h) or the all-day urine (24 h) of workers and DMF concentrations in the air (0-100 mg/m^3) in an artificial leather plant. The relationship was linear for the shift urine samples. For the 24-h urine samples, the relationship was linear only in the range of 0-80 mg DMF/m^3 (see also Table 10).

When Dixon et al. (1983) studied the urinary NMF excretion in a group of 32-37 workers who were exposed to similar air levels of DMF for either 8 h per shift (5 days/week) or 12 h per shift (4 days/week), they found higher concentrations of NMF in the urine when the workers were working 8-h shifts. A possible explanation was that a 13% reduction in urine volume was seen in workers on

8-h shifts during the summer months compared with higher urine outputs seen in the same workers on 12-h shifts during the winter months.

Sala et al. (1984) found a correlation between urinary NMF levels, 4 h after workplace exposure, and the workers' exposure levels to DMF in 5 job categories relating to artificial leather production. They reported airborne DMF concentrations of 4.5-14 mg/m^3 for spreading "coagulate" system workers, with a mean NMF in urine of 16 mg/g creatinine, 9.4 mg DMF/m^3 for finishing workers, with a mean NMF urinary value of 12 mg/g creatinine (low exposures), and 86.3 mg DMF/m^3 in tank cleaning workers with a corresponding urinary value of 188.3 mg NMF/g creatinine (highest exposure).

6.2.3.2 N,N-*Dimethylformamide determination in the expired air*

Airborne DMF concentrations change considerably during the work shift and from one workplace to another. Brugnone et al. (1980a) measured the DMF concentrations in the alveolar air every hour during the 8-h shift of 8 workers employed in an artificial leather plant. The alveolar DMF concentration in 6 workers was correlated with the DMF concentration in the air of the respective workplaces.

In a second study, Brugnone et al. (1984) studied 8 exposed workers by determining the DMF concentrations in the environmental air, alveolar air, blood, and urine. Air samples were collected at hourly intervals during an 8-h work shift, blood samples, at 2-h intervals, and urine samples, at 4-h intervals. No DMF was found in the blood or urine. A good correlation between the alveolar and environmental DMF concentrations was found in 6 out of the 8 workers, and at all subsequent hours, except for the fourth hour.

In practice, the alveolar air test is more difficult to perform and use for routine examination than measurement of NMF levels in urine samples, and is not recommended for biological monitoring.

6.2.3.3 Appraisal

The level of NMF in a post-shift urine sample is the most appropriate biological parameter for total DMF exposure (inhalation plus dermal) during the shift.

7. EFFECTS ON ORGANISMS IN THE ENVIRONMENT

The effects of DMF on organisms in the environment have been reviewed by Kennedy (1986) and by US EPA (1986).

The LC_{50}s of DMF for various aquatic species, given in Table 11, indicate a low toxicity for the species tested.

DMF is commonly used to facilitate the solution of lipophilic compounds in water during aquatic toxicity tests.

Cardwell et al. (1978) studied the long-term toxicity of DMF for fathead minnow *(Pimephales promelas)*, brown trout *(Salvelinus fontinalis)*, and bluegill *(Lepomis macrochirus)*, and found threshold limits of between 43 and 98 mg DMF/litre for the brook trout and between 5 and 10 mg/litre for the fathead minnow. LeBlanc & Surprenant (1983) showed that a level of 0.1 ml DMF/litre was acceptable for long-term aquatic toxicity tests. In a study by Tonogai et al. (1982), the 24-h and 48-h static median tolerance limits for the Himedaka *(Oryzias latipes)* were > 1000 mg DMF/litre.

Table 11. Medial lethal (LC_{50}) concentrations (mg/litre) for aquatic organisms exposed to dimethylformamide (DMF)

Species	LC_{50}			Reference
	24-h	48-h	96-h	
Guppy (*Paecilia reticulata*)	1300			Dojlido (1979)
Rainbow trout (*Salmo gairdneri*)			9800 9860	Poirier et al. (1986) Shubat et al. (1982)
Fathead minnow (*Pimephales promelas*)			10 600	Poirier et al. (1986)
Bluegill (*Lepomis macrochirus*)			7100	Poirier et al. (1986)
Midge (*Paratanytarsus parthenogeneticus*)		36 200		Poirier et al. (1986)
Daphnid (*Daphnia magna*)		14 500 12 300 (approx.)		Poirier et al. (1986) LeBlanc & Surprenant (1983)
Larvae (*Aedes aegypti*)		68 000 (approx.)		Kramer et al. (1983)

A no-observed-effect level (NOEL) of 7700 mg/litre was reported for the rainbow trout by Shubat et al. (1982).

Solutions of DMF of 25 g/litre (2.5%) were shown to be lethal within 0.5 h for eggs of sea urchins *(Lythechinus variegatus, Arbacia punctulata, Lythechinus pictus)*, the surf clam *(Spisule solidissima)*, and the annelid *(Pectinaria)* (Rebhun & Sawada, 1969).

Hughes & Vilkas (1983) determined that the highest concentration that had no significant effect on the green alga *Selenastrum capricornatum*, was 1 ml/litre and the no-effect level was 0.5 ml/litre.

Concentrations ranging from 0.085-0.340% DMF had an inhibitory effect on cultures of *Streptomyces aureofaciens* (Welward & Halama, 1978).

8. EFFECTS ON EXPERIMENTAL ANIMALS AND *IN VITRO* TEST SYSTEMS

8.1 Single exposures

Data on the acute toxicity of DMF in different laboratory animals, when administered by different routes, have been reviewed by Kennedy (1986). The acute toxicity in a number of species, following oral, dermal, inhalation (Table 12), or parenteral (Table 13) administration of DMF is relatively low, with lethal doses generally in the g/kg range for the oral, dermal, and parenteral routes and in the g/m^3 for inhalation exposures. Animals given large single doses of DMF or exposed to high air levels showed general depression, anaesthesia, loss of appetite, loss of body weight, tremors, laboured breathing, convulsions, haemorrhage of the nose and mouth, liver injury, and coma immediately preceding death.

In mice and rats, exposed to DMF via inhalation, signs of mucous membrane irritation were seen (Lobanova, 1958; Lundberg et al., 1986), and lung damage was detected histologically (Clayton et al., 1963).

Where tissue pathology was included in the study, the prominent organ showing damage was the liver (Massmann, 1956; Sanotsky et al., 1978; Mathew et al., 1980; Lundberg et al., 1981). No obvious species differences were observed with regard to acute lethality, but young rats appeared more sensitive to DMF-induced lethality than older rats (Kimura et al., 1971).

8.2 Skin and eye irritation, sensitization

DMF was reported to be irritating to the eyes, mucous membranes, and the skin (Hamilton & Hardy, 1974; Aldyreva & Gafurov, 1980).

8.2.1 Skin irritation

Rat tails dipped in DMF at 40 °C for 8 h became mummified in a few days (Massmann, 1956).

Table 12. LD_{50} and LC_{50} values of DMF after oral, dermal, or inhalation exposure in various animal species

Species	Oral LD_{50} (mg/kg)	Dermal LD_{50} (mg/kg)	Inhalation LC_{50} (mg/m³)	Reference
Rat	3000			Thiersch (1962)
			9432	US NIOSH (1977)
	3920			Massmann (1956)
		11 140		Schottek (1970, 1972)
	4000		12 000	Sanotsky et al. (1978)
		> 11 520		Bainova & Antov (1980)
			15 000	Clayton et al. (1963)
	4320			Lazarev & Levina (1976)
		11 000[a]		Stula & Krauss (1977)
			> 13 440	Lundberg et al. (1986)
	3200			Qin & Gue (1976)
			14 000	Cai & Huang (1979)
	7170			Bartsch et al. (1976)
Mouse	3950			Lazarev & Levina (1976)
	5550			Lazarev & Levina (1976)
		> 5000		Wiles & Narcisse (1971)
	6420		6000–9400	Bartsch et al. (1976)
	3700			Lobanova (1958)
	5400, 6200			Qin & Gue (1976)
			18 300	Cai & Huang (1979)
Rabbit	> 5000	> 500		Wiles & Narcisse (1971)
		1500[a]		Stula & Krauss (1977)
Mongolian gerbil	3929			Llewellyn et al. (1974)

[a] Pregnant females.

Table 13. LD$_{50}$s (mg/kg body weight) of DMF after parenteral administration in various animal species

Species	Intraperitoneal	Intravenous	Intramuscular	Subcutaneous	Reference
Rat	1480				Massmann (1956)
	2500				Thiersch (1962)
	4440				Bartsch et al. (1976)
	4600				Pham Huu Chanh et al. (1971)
	5470	2830	4030		Shottek (1970, 1972)
Mouse	300				Massmann (1956)
		3500	3800	4500	US NIOSH (1977)
	650				Barral-Chamaillard & Rouzioux (1983)
	1454				Burgun et al. (1975)
	2000				Antoine et al. (1983)
	3150	2800			Wiles & Narcisse (1971)
	5200				Pham Huu Chanh et al. (1971)
	5850	3490			Bartsch et al. (1976)
Rabbit	945	1800			Massmann (1956)
		1000			Wiles & Narcisse (1971)
	5000				US NIOSH (1977)
Guinea-pig	1300				Wahlberg & Boman (1979)
		1030			US NIOSH (1977)
	4000				Ungar et al. (1976)
Dog		470			Barral-Chamaillard & Rouzioux (1983)
Cat	500				Massmann (1956)

A single application of 500 mg DMF/kg resulted in transient irritation within 2-3 h in mice, but no irritation in rats (Wiles & Narcisse, 1971). DMF was slightly irritating for mice at doses of 2500 and 5000 mg/kg. No skin irritation was detected in rabbits with applications of 100, 200, or 500 mg DMF/kg. Single applications of DMF on the skin of rats and guinea-pigs did not cause irritation (Kiss, 1979; Bainova, 1985). Repeated 28-day treatments with 960 or 1920 mg/kg did not induce marked local dermal effects in rats (Bainova et al., 1985).

After repeated application of DMF to the skin of guinea-pigs for 21 days (Bainova, 1985), the mean irritative dose was 31% DMF (range 17-56%).

Dermal irritation was not seen in rabbits treated dermally with 2 g DMF/kg for 6 h, daily 15 times during a 4-week period (Kennedy, 1986).

8.2.2 Eye irritation

A 25% (25 g/litre) solution of DMF in water, injected into the conjunctival sac of the rabbit, did not produce any effects; 50% was slightly irritating, and 75-100% produced more severe irritation (Massmann, 1956). Single dose DMF instillation (0.1 ml) produced moderate corneal damage and conjunctival redness that was most pronounced at 2-3 days. By day 14, a mild degree of conjunctival redness, moderate corneal damage with an area of severe injury, slight surface distortion, and subsurface vascularization were observed (Kennedy & Sherman, 1986). In another study, the same authors reported that, after a single DMF instillation, the eye inflammation subsided and disappeared by the 8th day.

8.2.3 Sensitization

DMF was tested, using a maximization technique, on guinea-pigs to determine skin sensitization; it did not induce any response (Bainova, 1985).

Effects on animals and in vitro *test systems*

8.3 Repeated exposure

The effects of repeated oral, dermal, or inhalation exposure to DMF in various animal species have been reviewed by Kennedy (1986) and these data, together with other new information, are summarized in Table 14. In all species tested, except the dog, liver damage was produced, the degree of damage generally being proportional to the dose administered. In the two reported studies on the dog (Clayton et al., 1963; Kimmerle & Eben, 1975a), the inhalation exposure conditions appeared to be too low (60 mg/m^3) to produce damage, though 1 out of the 4 dogs tested by Clayton did have altered liver function tests. Higher levels were not tested. Some evidence of recovery from the hepatotoxic effects of DMF was found in rats (Kennedy & Sherman, 1986).

Higher, intermittent doses of DMF appeared to produce more pronounced effects in male rats than continuous dosing (Bainova et al., 1981a; Bainova, 1985). Tanaka (1971) found more pronounced liver damage in rats following one rather than three weeks of exposure and considered that the high regenerative capacity of liver tissue was responsible for the observation.

Other tissues and organs that are affected, particularly by high doses of DMF, will be discussed in section 8.4.

8.4 Specific organ toxicity

8.4.1 Liver

The potency of DMF as a hepatotoxic agent has been reviewed by Kennedy (1986) and by Scailteur & Lauwerys (1987). The effects of DMF on the liver were studied after single or repeated inhalation, dermal, or oral treatment of rats, mice, and rabbits (Massmann, 1956; Clayton et al., 1963; Shottek, 1970; Tanaka, 1971; Kimmerle & Eben, 1975a; Medyankin, 1975; Sanotsky et al., 1978; Germanova et al., 1979; Mathew et al., 1980; Bainova et al., 1981a; Lundberg et al., 1981; Lundberg, 1982; Brondeau et al., 1983; Bainova, 1985; Kennedy & Sherman, 1986; Scailteur & Lauwerys, 1987). Single oral administrations of 2250-5000 mg DMF/kg in rats (Kennedy &

Table 14. Effects of repeated oral, dermal, or inhalation exposure to DMF in various animal species

Species	Route of exposure	Dose	Duration	Effects	Reference
Mongolian gerbil	oral	10 000 mg/kg drinking-water	30 days	no changes in body weight, liver, or kidney	Llewellyn et al. (1974)
		10 000 mg/kg drinking-water	200 days	mortality in 25% of animals; liver necrosis	
		17 000 mg/kg drinking-water	80 days	mortality with liver necrosis; LD_{50} cumulative 90 206 mg/kg body weight	
		34 000 mg/kg drinking-water	6 days	mortality with liver necrosis; LD_{50} cumulative 3846 mg/kg body weight	
Mouse	oral	620 or 1240 mg/kg diet	30 days	anorexia, loss of body weight	Qin & Gue (1976)
		160, 540, 1850 mg/kg diet	119 days	dose-related increase in relative and absolute liver weights; no other histological or biochemical changes; NOEL, 246-326 mg/kg diet per day	Becci et al. (1983)
Rat	oral	320 or 640 mg/kg diet	30 days	anorexia, loss of body weight	Qin & Gue (1976)
		50, 500, 5000 mg/litre drinking-water	100 days	body weight decrease; liver damage at 5000 mg/litre; increase in liver to body weight ratio at 500 and 5000 mg/litre; structural liver changes and regeneration at 5000 mg/litre; NOEL, 50 mg/litre	Qin & Gue (1976)

Table 14 (continued)

Species	Route of exposure	Dose	Duration	Effects	Reference
Rat	oral	102, 497, 1000 mg/litre drinking-water	14 days 49 days	no behavioural changes at 102 or 497 mg/litre for 49 days; dose-related deviations in cerebral and glial cell enzyme activities	Savolainen (1981)
		215, 750, 2500 mg/kg diet	104 days	dose-related increase in relative and absolute liver weights, considered to be physiological adaptation; NOEL, 210-235 mg/kg diet per day	Becci et al. (1983)
		200, 1000, 5000 mg/kg diet (equivalent to 12, 60, 300 mg/kg/body weight per day)	90 days	slight anaemia and leukocytosis, hypercholesterolaemia at 1000 and 5000 mg/kg diet; NOEL, 200 mg/kg diet	Kennedy & Sherman (1986)
		0.1, 0.5, 1.0 g/litre in drinking-water	14 days 49 days	dose-related increase in liver/body weight ratios; in liver and kidneys, increased values of reduced glutathione, microsomal UDP glucuronosyl transferase, and ethoxycoumarin O-demethylase activities; no changes in liver microsomal cytochrome P-450 or ADPH-cytochrome reductase activity	Elovaara et al. (1983)
Rat	dermal	470 mg/kg per day for 29 days and 11 140 mg/kg on the 30th day	30 days	continuous dosing caused hepatotoxicity and did not protect against lethality; pretreatment did not enhance toxic reactions after application of the LD_{50} in 30-day pretreated rats	Schottek (1970)
		215, 430, 960, or 4800 mg/kg per day	30 days	dose-related changes in GOT, GPT, AlcP, ChE, gamma-GT, lipid fractions in serum and liver homogenates; NOEL, 215 mg/kg	Bainova & Antov (1980)

Table 14 (continued)

Rat	dermal	215, 320, 960, or 4800 mg/kg per day	30 days	dose-related changes (at doses > 320 mg/kg) in enzyme activities in liver, myocardium, and kidney homogenates; NOEL, 215 mg/kg	Bainova (1985)
Rat	dermal	960 mg/kg daily or 1920 mg/kg applied intermittently[a]	28 days	functional, biochemical, and pathomorphological changes in liver; and lipid metabolism on the 4th, 8th, 14th, and 28th day of the tests; changes more pronounced after intermittent exposure	Bainova et al. (1981a) Bainova (1985)
		4-h dipping of tails in 60, 65, 70, or 80% DMF in water	60 days	concentration-related changes in liver and nervous system; NOEL, 60% DMF in water	Medyankin (1975)
		4-h dipping of tails in 30 or 60% DMF and inhalation of 5 or 10 mg DMF/m^3, 6 h daily	120 days	no changes at 30% DMF contact and 5 mg DMF/m^3 inhalation; adverse effects at other concentrations	Medyankin (1975)
Rabbit	dermal	50, 100% water solution, 3 times/day, 2 ml/application	7 days	died at 5-8 day of application at 100% DMF; liver biochemical and histological changes	Huang et al. (1981)
		2000 mg/kg per day	9 days	anorexia, cyanosis, and mortality with liver necrosis	Kennedy & Sherman (1986)
Guinea-pig	dermal	50, 75, 100% solution, 3 times/day 2 ml/application	7 days	died 2-4 days after application of 75 or 100% and 4-9 days after 50%; loss of body weight; liver damage	Huang et al. (1981)

Table 14 (continued)

Species	Route of exposure	Dose	Duration	Effects	Reference
Rat	inhalation	1800 mg/m³ for 6 h daily	6 days	concentration-related mortality; cumulation of hepatoxic effect	Schottek (1970)
		750 and 1500 mg/m³, 6 h daily	6 days		
		30 mg/m³ for 6 h daily	8 days	no changes in the function of the thyroid or adrenal glands	Sanotsky & Ulanova (1975)
		aerosol for 0.5 h daily (concentration unknown)	3 or 30 days	liver and kidney necrosis, lung changes, arterial changes in myocardium	Santa Cruz & Corpino (1978); Santa Cruz & Maccioni (1978)
		22 ± 1.6 mg/m³ for 6 h daily, 6 days a week	18 weeks	liver changes, no other responses	Cai & Huang (1979)
Rat	inhalation	130 mg/m³ for 4 h daily	27 days	functional changes in kidneys and liver; arterial blood pressure more pronounced after additional single administration of 500 mg DMF/kg on the 1st, 8th, and 27th days of the studies, and after intermittent exposure	Germanova et al. (1979)
		300 mg/m³ in 5 peaks of 15 min at 40-min intervals	27 days		
		7569 mg/m³ for 6 h daily	5 days	weakness, weight loss, dehydration, liver necrosis	Kennedy & Sherman (1986)
Young rat (3-12 weeks old)	inhalation	600 mg/m³ for 8 h daily	28 days	increased serum GOT and GPT; morphological liver changes, mainly in 3-week-old rats; no histological abnormalities in other organs	Tanaka (1971)

Table 14 (continued)

Species	Route	Dose	Duration	Effects	Reference
Young rat (3 weeks old)	inhalation	600 mg/m³ for 8 h daily and 600 mg/m³ for 1 h daily	28 days	liver changes at the 1st, 2nd, 3rd, and 4th week of test more intense in the group exposed for 8 h daily; no cumulation of hepatoxic effect	Tanaka (1971)
Rat, mouse	inhalation	450, 900, 1800, 3600 mg/m³ for 6 h daily	60 days	increased serum GOT, GPT, AlcP, cholesterol, anaemia and histological liver changes at 900 mg/m³ or more; liver weight increase at 450 mg/m³; NOEL below 450 mg/m³ in both species	Craig et al. (1984)
Rat, cat	inhalation	300, 690, 1350 mg/m³, 8 h daily	120 days	anorexia, weight loss, liver degeneration, and necrosis; changes in brain, myocardium, and kidneys; no abnormalities in blood tests or ECG	Massmann (1956)
Rabbit	inhalation	22 ± 1.6 mg/m³ for 6 h daily, 6 days per week	18 weeks	no changes in ECG or liver parameters	Cai & Huang (1979)
		317 ± 37.8 mg/m³ for 6 h daily, 6 days a week	14 weeks	body weight changes; liver damage functionally and structurally; by congestion and haemorrhage	Cai & Huang (1979)
		120 mg/m³ for 8 h daily	50 days	microscopic and electronmicroscopic changes in the myocardium	Arena et al. (1982)
Dog	inhalation	60 mg/m³ for 6 h daily	107 days	reversible changes in blood pressure, ECG, and in liver functions	Clayton et al. (1963)
		63 mg/m³ for 6 h daily	28 days	normal GOT, GPT, bilirubin, urea, and creatinine in plasma; NOEL, 63 mg DMF/m³	Kimmerle & Eben (1975a)

[a] Two alternative intermittent regimes were used: (i) 1920 mg/kg per day for 2 days, followed by no treatment for 2 days; (ii) 1920 mg/kg every second day.

Sherman, 1986) caused clay-coloured liver, congestion, and centrilobular necrosis of hepatocytes. Lower doses resulted in deviations in liver function, such as decreased excretion of cholic acid in the bile, bromosulfthalein retention, increased serum activities of GOT, GPT, LAP, OCT, AlcP, ChE, LDH, and gamma-GT, and significant enhancement of cholesterol, triglyceride, and bilirubin contents in the serum and liver homogenates. In rats, following both intraperitoneal (ip) and inhalation exposure, there were no increases in SDH levels at 420 and 840 mg/m^3 but a lower level (210 mg/m^3) raised the serum activity of SDH (Lundberg et al., 1986). Pathomorphological investigation demonstrated lipid degeneration and cloudy swelling of hepatocytes in the central zones of the lobules followed by signs of regeneration.

DMF at 0.6 ml/kg, administered intraperitoneally, caused mild changes in rat liver lobules. Marked centrilobular necrosis and central phlebitis were found in the rats treated with single ip doses of 0.9 and 1.2 ml DMF/kg (Mathew et al., 1980). A single ip dose of 0.5 ml DMF/kg to hamsters caused centrilobular necrosis accompanied by haemosiderosis (Ungar et al., 1976). Morphological changes were reported in the liver by Clayton et al. (1963), Shottek (1970), Tanaka (1971), and Santa Cruz & Corpino (1978) after repeated DMF exposure of young animals, with periodic peaks (Table 14).

Diets supplemented with DMF at levels of 215, 750, or 2500 mg/kg for 104 days for rats and 160, 540, or 1850 mg/kg for 119 days for mice, resulted in significant dose-related increases in relative liver weights in all experimental animals. No deviations were reported in the serum activities of GOT, GPT, AlcP, other than an increase in GPT activity in mice fed a diet containing 1850 mg DMF/kg. Histopathological evaluation did not reveal any hepatotoxicity (Becci et al., 1983). The oral administration of a 10% water solution of DMF (400 mg/kg body weight) for 14 days (Leshik & Feoktistova, 1984) to guinea-pigs significantly decreased the ascorbic acid content and the concentration of cytochrome P-450 in the liver. The daily intake of 0.1, 0.5, or 1.0 g DMF/litre in the drinking-water for 2 or 7 weeks (Elovaara et al., 1983) increased the liver/body weight ratios, the microsomal UDP-glucuronosyl-transferase and 7-ethoxycoumarin-O-demethylase activity, and reduced the glutathione concentration in liver homogenates.

No liver injury was seen following inhalation exposure of dogs to 63 mg DMF/m^3 (Kimmerle & Eben, 1975a). However, in another study, 1 out of 4 dogs exposed to 60 mg/m^3 showed increased enzyme values (Clayton et al., 1963)). Liver injury was also not seen: after inhalation exposure of rats at levels of < 450 mg/m^3 (Craig et al., 1984), after dermal exposure of rats at a level of 240 mg/kg (Bainova, 1985), and at dietary levels of 215 mg/kg body weight per day for rats and 160 mg/kg for mice (Becci et al., 1983).

8.4.2 Gastrointestinal tract

Toxic gastroenteritis with pathomorphological deviations was described in the experimental animals treated at high doses or concentrations in studies reported in Table 14 (Massmann, 1956; Clayton et al., 1963; Shottek, 1970).

8.4.3 Cardiovascular system

Microscopic examination did not reveal any myocardial lesions in rats and mice after ingestion of dietary levels of 215, 750, or 2500 mg DMF/kg for 104 days, or 160, 540, or 1850 mg DMF/kg for 119 days, respectively (Becci et al., 1983).

Clayton et al. (1963) and Germanova et al. (1979) reported decreases in blood pressure in dogs (not cats) following exposure to DMF. The changes described were not great and, in the absence of confirmatory data in other test models (and in man), are of questionable significance. Large iv doses (500 mg/kg) did not produce any changes in the contractile force of myocardial tissue in dogs (Pham Huu Chanh et al., 1973).

Santa Cruz & Maccioni (1978) described histological changes in the myocardium of the rat and Clayton et al. (1963) described subtle blood pressure changes in the dog. The findings in the rat followed high exposures; the blood pressure changes in the dog were minimal and hard to differentiate from those in control animals.

8.4.4 Kidney

Swelling of the kidney tubules occurred after a single oral administration of 2250-5000 mg DMF/kg in rats (Kennedy &

Sherman, 1986). Short-term feeding studies in rats and mice (Table 14) did not reveal any histopathological lesions in the kidneys (Becci et al., 1983; Kennedy & Sherman, 1986).

A number of pathomorphological studies revealed vacuolar degeneration, mainly in the renal tubules (Massmann, 1956; Clayton et al., 1963; Santa Cruz & Corpino, 1978; Lundberg et al., 1983). Costa et al. (1978) observed histological, histochemical, and electron-microscopic renal lesions in groups of rats, exposed to DMF aerosols (dose not stated) for 1 h/day for 15 days or for 0.5 h/day for 30 days. Degeneration took place in the proximal part of tubules and in the visceral epithelium of the glomerulus with marked mitochondrial changes.

Repeated inhalation exposure to 130 or 300 mg DMF/m^3 increased the kidney/body weight ratio, and decreased diuresis, and the total protein, sodium chloride, and potassium contents in the urine of rats (Germanova et al., 1979).

Elovaara et al. (1983) reported enhanced activities of 7-ethoxy-coumarin-O-demethylase, and UDP-glucuronosyltransferase, and a decrease in cytosolic formaldehyde dehydrogenase activity in rats orally exposed to DMF. Bainova & Antov (1980) and Bainova et al. (1981b) reported that the 30-day dermal application of 960 or 4800 mg DMF/kg resulted in dose-related increased activities of SucDH, G-6-PDH, and LDH in rat kidney homogenates.

8.4.5 Nervous system

Functional changes in the nervous system were observed after administration of high doses or exposure to high concentrations of DMF (Massmann, 1956; Clayton et al., 1963) and after prolonged treatment with moderate doses of DMF (Medyankin, 1975; Sanotsky et al., 1978; Germanova et al., 1979; Bainova, 1985) (Table 14). Doses within the range of lethal levels resulted in anaesthesia, depression, or coma. Moderate doses caused inhibition of motor activity.

No effects on the behaviour of rats were noted after they drank DMF in the drinking-water for 2 and 7 weeks at doses ranging from 1.4 to 13.7 mmol/litre with a cumulative dose of 3200 mg/kg in the rats (Savolainen, 1981). The same dose enhanced the activities of acid proteinase and 2,3-cyclicnucleotide-3'-phosphohydrolase in the glial cells.

Massmann (1956) and Clayton et al. (1963) observed pathomorphological changes in the brains of experimental animals after treatment with high doses of DMF (Table 14).

8.4.6 Lungs

Lung congestion and oedema were found in rats after single oral application of 2250-5000 mg DMF/kg (Kennedy & Sherman, 1986).

Bronchopneumonic changes were observed in experimental animals after inhalation of high DMF concentrations (Massmann, 1956; Clayton et al., 1963; Shottek, 1970; Santa Cruz & Corpino, 1978) (Table 14). According to the authors, the changes were related to injury of the small arterial vessels and, to some extent, to local irritation caused by DMF.

8.4.7 Haematopoietic system

High levels of DMF might cause some anaemia, but no other changes in the erythrocytes of experimental animals have been reported (Massmann, 1956; Clayton et al., 1963; Sanotsky et al., 1978; Germanova et al., 1979; Bainova & Antov, 1980) (Table 14). Depressed bone marrow activity was reported in rats after a single oral administration of 2250-5000 mg DMF/kg (Kennedy & Sherman, 1986). Pham Huu Chanh et al. (1971) found leukocytosis in rats after repeated ip injections of DMF.

Pathomorphological changes were observed in the spleen after exposure to high doses of DMF. They were accompanied by an increase in the spleen/body weight ratio (Massmann, 1956; Clayton et al., 1963; Bainova & Antov, 1980; Bainova, 1985). Medyankin (1975) found inhibited phagocytosis activity of leukocytes and decreased glycogen content in the neutrophiles of rats as a result of combined dermal and inhalation exposure to DMF.

8.4.8 Adrenals

Clayton et al. (1963) observed histological changes in the adrenal glands after inhalation of DMF. Decreased ascorbic acid content in the adrenals of rats was reported by Germanova et al. (1979), during intermittent and continuous inhalation exposure to DMF (Table 14).

8.4.9 Gonads

Male rats were exposed to 584-616 mg DMF/m^3 or 49-51 mg/m^3 for 4 h daily for 2, 4, or 8 days; female rats were exposed to 2.3 or 10.7 mg DMF/m^3, for 4 h daily, for 30 days (Sheveleva et al., 1979). Examination of the sperm and the histological study of the testes and ovaries did not show any pathological signs.

Lewis et al. (1979) exposed male rats at 90 or 900 mg DMF/m^3, for 6 h daily, over 5 days. Gross and histological examination of the testes did not reveal any pathological changes.

The histological examination of male rats, treated orally in short-term studies (Becci et al., 1983; Kennedy & Sherman, 1986) with a variety of doses (Table 14), did not result in changes in the testes. No lesions were noted in the male rats after a 30-day dermal application of DMF (Bainova, 1985). Craig et al. (1984) did not find testicular or ovarian lesions in rats and mice after short-term inhalation exposure to DMF at concentrations of up to 3600 mg/m^3 (Table 14).

Examination of the gonads in a large number of the acute and repeated-dose toxicity studies discussed earlier did not reveal them to be a target for DMF toxicity.

8.5 Developmental toxicity and reproduction

DMF was investigated for developmental toxicity in mice, rats, and rabbits using the oral, dermal, and inhalation routes and parenteral injection. According to present-day requirements, most of the older studies were not adequately designed or described. A survey is given in Tables 15, 16, 17.

No 3-generation reproduction studies were available.

Table 15. DMF administration to pregnant mice

Route	Dose[a]	Maternal toxicity	Embryotoxicity	Malformations	Reference
Gavage	control 193 µl/kg (gavage; day 6-15 pc)	-	fetal weights decreased	4 of 245 living fetuses showed malformations	Hellwig et al. (in press)
	580 µl/kg (gavage; day 6-15 pc)	NR[b]	fetal weights decreased	17 of 241 living fetuses showed malformations	
Intra-peritoneal injection	control 170 mg/kg (day 1-14 pc)	- NR[b]	- -	- -	Scheufler & Freye (1975)
	250 mg/kg (day 6-14 pc)	NR[b]	-	-	
	600 mg/kg 1100 mg/kg (day 1-14 pc)	NR[b]	late resorptions	malformation rates 18 and 75% respectively	
Intra-peritoneal injection	0.4 mg/kg (day 11-15 pc) 1.0 mg/kg (day 11-15 pc)	- +	- 2/6 abortions	- 8/36 malformations	Hellwig et al. (in press)

[a] pc = Post conception.
[b] NR = Not reported.

Table 16. DMF administration to pregnant rats

Route	Dose[a]	Maternal toxicity	Embryotoxicity	Malformations	Reference
Gavage	control 176 µl/kg (day 6-15 pc)	-	-	-	Hellwig et al. (in press)
	533 µl/kg	-	some embryo-lethality in the early phase, reduced fetal weights + retardations + variations	+	
	1600 µl/kg	weight stationary between day 6-15	63% embryo-lethality in the median phase	12% of the 85 living fetuses were malformed	
Dermal	day 6-10 and 13-15 pc				Hellwig et al. (in press)
	0 µl/kg	-	-	-	
	100 µl/kg	-	-	2.46%	
	500 µl/kg	-	-	3.05%	
	1000 µl/kg	-	slight reduced fetal length	5.46% (increase in rib and vertebral abnormalities)	

Table 16 (continued)

Dermal					Stula & Krauss (1977)
	control 600 mg/kg (days 9, 10 + 11, 11 + 12, 12 + 13 pc)	reduced weight gain	-	-	
	1200 mg/kg (day 10 + 11 pc)	reduced weight gain	slight embryolethality		
	1200 mg/kg (day 12 + 13 pc)	reduced weight gain	slight embryolethality	-	
	2400 mg/kg (day 10 + 11 pc)	stationary weight	embryolethality	-	
	400 or 200 mg/kg (applied 6 times/day days 11 + 12 + 13 pc)	reduced weight gain	high embryo-lethality	-	
			slight	embryolethality	

Table 16 (continued)

Route	Dose[a]	Maternal toxicity	Embryotoxicity	Malformations	Reference
Inhalation	control	-	-	-	Hellwig et al. (in press)
	861 mg/m³ (287 ppm) (day 0-1, 4-8, 11-15, 18-19 pc)	reduced weight gain	reduced fetal weights resorptions	-	
	861 mg/m³ (287 ppm) (day 0-3, 6-10, 13-18 pc)	reduced weight gain	reduced fetal weights retardations resorptions variations	-	
	660 mg/m³ (220 ppm) (day 4-8 pc)	-	reduced weight and length	-	
	1560 mg/m³ (520 ppm) (day 4-8 pc)	reduced weight gain	embyro-lethality; reduced weights	-	
Inhalation	control	-	-	-	Kimmerele & Machemer (1975)
	54 mg/m³ (18 ppm)	-	-	-	
	516 mg/m³ (172 ppm) (6-15 day pc)	-	reduced fetal weights	-	

Table 16 (continued)

Inhalation	control 96 mg/m³ (32 ppm) 903 mg/m³ (301 ppm) (day 6-15 pc)	– – reduced weight gain	– – ossification variations slightly increased from 60 to 75%	Keller & Lewis (1981)
Inhalation	control 1200 mg/m³ (400 ppm) (4 h/day, 10-20 day pc)	– NR	– total resorptions in some animals, no retardations	Shottek (1964)
Inhalation	0.05 mg/litre ~48 mg/m³ (~16 ppm) (day 0-20 pc)	NR	weight decrease	Sheveleva & Osina (1973)
Inhalation	0.8 mg/litre ~600 mg/m³ (~200 ppm)	NR	embryolethality; weight decrease	
Intravenous injection	control 0.5 g/kg on days 10, 11, or 12 pc	– NR	– –	Parkie & Webb (1983)

[a] pc = Post conception.
[b] NR = Not reported.

Table 17. DMF administration to pregnant rabbits

Route	Dose[a]	Maternal toxicity	Embryotoxicity	Malformations	Reference
Gavage	control	-	-	-	Merkle & Zeller (1980)
	46.4 μl/kg (day 6-18 pc)	-	-	1 hydrocephalus	
	68.1 μl/kg (day 6-18 pc)	-	decrease in number of implantations and % living implantations	3 hydrocephalus	
	200 μl/kg (day 8-16 pc)	decrease in food intake, weight gain, and placental weight	decrease in fetal weight, 3 abortions, placental weight decrease	+ 16 fetuses in 7 litters were malformed:	
Dermal	control	-	-	-	Stula & Krauss (1977)
	200 mg/kg day 8-16 pc		some embryolethality	-	
Dermal	control 100 mg/kg per day; semi-occlusive (day 6-28 pc)	-	-	1.1% fetuses per litter skeletal anomalies; 3.3% agenesia of gall bladder	Hellwig et al. (in press)

Table 17 (continued)

Dermal (continued)	200 mg/kg per day	-	-	
	400 mg/kg per day	decrease in body weight on day 16 and 18	-	23.5% fetuses per litter sternal anomalies; 2.45% hernia umbilicalis, 6.08% agenesia of gall bladder	Hellwig et al. (in press)
Inhalation	Control 150 mg/m³ (50 ppm) (day 7-19 pc)	-	-	-	
	450 mg/m³ (150 ppm)	decrease in body weight gain	increase in sternal variations	1 hernia umbilicalis (50 fetuses)	
	1350 mg/m³ (450 ppm)	decrease in body weight gain	decrease in weights, increase in variations (pseudoankylosis)	incidence of hernia umbilicalis increased; skeletal and soft tissue anomalies	

ᵃ pc = Post conception.

8.5.1 Developmental toxicity

8.5.1.1 Mouse

Administration by gavage of 580 or 193 µl DMF/kg per day, from day 6 to 15 after conception, to 26 mice per dose group led to a dose-dependent decrease in fetal weights and an increase in the number of retardations and variations. At 580 µl/kg per day, 17 out of 241 fetuses were malformed (cleft palate, exencephaly, hydrocephalus internus, aplasia of presphenoid). No maternal effects were recorded; the number of live fetuses remained unchanged. At 193 µl/kg, 4 out of 245 fetuses showed malformations. In untreated control groups for each dose group, 2 out of 229 and 1 out of 310 fetuses, respectively, had a cleft palate (Hellwig et al., in press).

After an ip injection of 600 or 1100 mg DMF/kg per day, from day 1 to 14 after conception, embryotoxic and teratogenic effects were registered. The malformation rates were 18 and 75%, respectively, and the effects consisted of absence or retardation of posterior skull ossification, open eye-lids, cerebral oedema, sternal haematomas, and spina bifida-like defects in the thoracic region. Embryotoxic effects recorded were late resorptions. Doses of 170 mg/kg per day from day 1 to 14 after conception, and 250 mg/kg per day from day 6-14, and single doses of 2100 mg/kg each on days 3, 7, 9, or 11 after conception, did not produce any effects (Scheufler & Freye, 1975).

In another ip injection study on mice, 6 animals per dose group were treated with 0.4 or 1.0 mg DMF/kg per day from day 11 to 15 after conception. Maternal body weight gain was reduced at 1.0 mg/kg per day, 2 out of 6 animals had abortions, 7 out of 36 fetuses showed exencephaly and 1 had a cleft palate. No effects were observed at 0.4 mg/kg (Hellwig et al., in press).

The studies indicate that DMF may be teratogenic for mice.

8.5.1.2 Rat

In a gavage study on groups of 26 rats administered 1600 µl DMF/kg per day from day 6 to 15 after conception, maternal toxicity was observed in the form of decreased body weight. Sixty-three percent of the implantations were resorbed and 12% of the surviving 85 (36.64%) fetuses were malformed (9 cases of diffuse anasarca, 2 cases of tail aplasia, 1 micrognathia, furthermore several fetuses had anomalies of the ribs, sternum, and vertebral column). A dose of 533 μl DMF/kg per day caused some early fetal deaths, in the absence of clinical signs of maternal toxicity, reduced fetal weight, and also some malformations, as well as an increase in variations and skeletal retardations. The malformations consisted of: 2 cases of tail aplasia, 2 cases of cleft palate, 1 atresia ani, 1 anasarca, 1 open eye, and several fetuses with split and aplastic vertebrae. At 176 μl/kg, decreased placental weights and some decreases in fetal length and increases in fetal weight were seen. All other parameters were within the range of biological variability (Hellwig et al., in press).

The dermal studies on rats did not fulfil today's criteria for a valid study.

In one series of studies (Hellwig et al., in press), 0, 100, 500, or 1000 μl DMF/kg per day (undiluted material) were administered in an uncovered dermal system from day 6 to 10 and then from day 13 to 15 after conception (26 animals per dose group; 10 in the control group). Under these conditions, 1000 μl/kg per day caused a slightly retarded weight gain among the dams and significant dermal irritation. The fetuses were slightly smaller. Malformations consisted of split thoracic vertebrae and anomalies of the ribs. The rate of the malformations in live fetuses was 0% per litter in the controls and 2.46%, 3.05%, and 5.46% with increasing dose level. This may indicate a weak dose-related teratogenic effect.

In another study (Stula & Krauss, 1977), rats received dermal doses of up to 2400 mg (undiluted DMF)/kg per day, at least every 2 days, from day 9 to 13 after conception, under non-occlusive conditions. There was clear evidence of embryolethality at 2400 mg/kg per day on gestation days 10 and 11 (26%, i.e., 7 rats) and at 1200 and 2400 mg/kg per day (in 6 portions of 200 and 400 mg) on gestation days 11, 12, and 13 with incidences of 43 and 30%, respectively. Maternal weight gain and average fetal weights were also suppressed. Fetal abnormalities were not observed, with the exception of a few subcutaneous haematomas, which occurred at a rate also seen in historical controls at this laboratory.

Several inhalation studies were carried out on rats. In one study, 23 animals per dose group were exposed to 54 or 516 mg DMF/m^3 (18 or 172 ppm) over 6 h per day from day 6 to 15 after conception. There were 22 animals in the control group. The higher exposure level caused a decrease in fetal weights in the absence of signs of maternal toxicity. No effects were seen on the numbers of implantations, resorption rates, placental weights, number of fetuses weighing less than 3 g (runts), variations in skeletal development or malformations; the lower exposure level (54 mg/m^3) did not cause any adverse effects (Kimmerle & Machemer, 1975).

In another rat study, exposure to 903 mg/m^3 (301 ppm) for 6 h per day, from day 6 to 15 after conception (19 animals per group) led to a reduction in maternal weight gain and to a slightly increased incidence of skeletal (ossification) variations of from 60 to 75%. Exposure to 96 mg/m^3 (32 ppm) did not produce any effect (Keller & Lewis, 1981).

Following 10 exposures to 1200 mg/m^3 (400 ppm) for 4 h per day, from day 10 to 20 after conception, dead implants (54% total resorptions compared with 15% in the controls) occurred. The numbers of animals in the treated and control groups were not reported (Shottek, 1964).

Fetal weight decreases and fetal deaths were reported in another study on rats after exposure to 600 mg/m^3 (200 ppm) from day 0 throughout the gestation period. Exposure to 48 mg/m^3 (16 ppm) was said to have caused reduced fetal weights. However, the description of the study was inadequate (Sheveleva & Osina, 1973).

A series of inhalation studies on rats is described (Hellwig et al., in press) in which the exposure periods did not fully cover the critical period of the gestation phase (e.g., "window dosing" or non-exposure during weekends, see Table 17). In one set of these experiments, exposure to concentrations of 660 and 1560 mg/m^3 (220 and 520 ppm), for 6 h per day (days 0-3, 6-10, 11-18 after conception; 18 animals per group) caused decreased fetal weights, retardations, and an increase in embryolethality. Another exposure regimen, i.e., 861 mg/m^3 (287 ppm), for 6 h per day, was administered on days 1, 4-8, 11-15, and 18-19 after conception to a group of 30 rats. Twenty animals were subjected to caesarian section on day 20 after conception, the offsprings of the other 10 animals were raised until day 21 after birth. Thirty rats served as untreated controls. There was retarded maternal weight gain from the beginning of the treatment; fetal weights were decreased, and the numbers of variations and retardations were increased. No malformations were found.

No effects were detected after single iv injections of 0.5 g/kg body weight between days 10, 11, or 12 after conception (Parkie & Webb, 1983). Furthermore, earlier investigations on rats after single ip or sc injections did not give any indication of teratogenicity; however, such studies are of limited value for a toxicity assessment.

The above studies indicate that DMF is embryotoxic in the rat. After dermal and oral administration, teratogenicity may also occur.

8.5.1.3 Rabbit

DMF caused maternal toxicity and embryotoxicity, including teratogenicity, in rabbits after administration by gavage at 200 µl/kg per day from day 6-18 after conception. All 11 animals in the dose group became pregnant and showed reduced food intake and weight gain. Placental weights were significantly lower and 3 abortions occurred. The fetuses showed weight reduction. The main findings recorded on fetal examination were hernia umbilicalis (7 cases), hydrocephalus internus (6 cases), eventratio simplex (3 cases), exophthalmus (2 cases), cleft palate (1 case), and malposition of limbs (1 case). The number of implantations was not adversely influenced. At 68.1 µl/kg per day, no maternal effects were observed among 16 pregnant animals (18 inseminated); decreased numbers of total implantations and of live fetuses occurred, also an increase in skeletal variations and retardations per litter; 3 cases of hydrocephalus internus were present. At 46.4 µl/kg per day (10/12 does were pregnant) 1 case of hydrocephalus internus occurred; all other parameters were in the range of biological variability. No malformations occurred in the untreated control group (22/24 animals) (Merkle & Zeller, 1980).

In a dermal study, 5 rabbits (4 animals in the control group) received 200 mg DMF/kg per day, dermally, from day 8 to day 16 after conception. The test material was applied in undiluted form on the intact skin, apparently under non-occlusive conditions. Embryo mortality was 6% compared with 3% in the controls. The average fetal weight was 32.9 g in the litters of treated animals compared with 28.4 g among controls. Fetal abnormalities were not detected (Stula & Krauss, 1977).

In another dermal study (Hellwig et al., in press), dose levels of undiluted DMF of 0, 100, 200, or 400 mg/kg per day were applied for 6 h/day, under semi-occlusive conditions (15 animals per dose group). A 5-6% decrease in maternal body weights occurred in the highest dose group, towards the end of the treatment period (days 16-18 after conception). At this dose level, an increase in skeletal (sternal) malformations was found in 15 fetuses in 7 litters investigated (23.5%), and also 5 cases of missing gall bladder (in 2 litters). No malformations occurred in animals in the 200 mg/kg per day group or in the untreated control group. At 100 mg/kg per day, one fetus had a sternal anomaly, 2 fetuses had gall bladder agenesis, and one of the latter a hypertrophic-dilatative cardiac-aortic malformation.

In a recent inhalation study, exposure levels were 0, 150, 450, and 1350 mg/m^3 (0, 50, 150, and 450 ppm) over 6 h per day from day 7 to day 19 after conception (fifteen animals per dose group). Animals in the highest exposure group showed a slight retardation in body weight gain as a sign of maternal toxicity. The fetal weights were significantly lower in this group, and there was a significant increase in malformations, mostly hernia umbilicalis (7 out of 86 fetuses, in 4 out of 15 litters) and some soft-tissue malformations, such as missing gall bladder, without statistical significance. In addition, anomalies of the sternum, an increase in split vertebrae, and a number of variations were also recorded. At 450 mg/m^3, maternal body weights were slightly retarded during the exposure period and the corrected body weight gain was marginally, but significantly, decreased. One case of hernia umbilicalis among 75 fetuses and an increase in sternal variations were observed. At 150 mg/m^3, neither fetuses nor does showed any indications of response to treatment. In summary, signs of embryotoxicity and teratogenicity were seen at the highest concentration (1350 mg/m^3) and to a lesser degree at 450 mg/m^3. The maternal toxicity seen at 1350 mg/m^3 and 450 mg/m^3 is in accordance with the maternal toxicity observed at 900 mg/m^3 in a previous range-finding study (Hellwig et al., in press).

These studies indicate that DMF may be teratogenic for rabbits.

3.5.1.4 Appraisal

The overall conclusion from all studies is that DMF may lead to embryotoxic and teratogenic effects in rats, mice, and rabbits. An increase in malformations in the absence of maternal toxicity is clearly visible after gavage and ip administration, with a smaller incidence after dermal administration. In general, the rabbit appeared to be more sensitive to the teratogenic effects of DMF than the rat. After inhalation exposure, fetal toxicity and teratogenic effects appear to be confined to conditions of maternal toxicity.

8.6 Mutagenicity and related end-points

DMF has been tested extensively in mutagenicity and genotoxicity assays. DMF was one of the 42 chemicals selected for study in the International Collaborative Program for the Evaluation of Short-Term Tests for Carcinogens (Serres & Ashby, 1981).

The genetic toxicity studies on DMF have been reviewed by Purchase et al. (1978), Kennedy (1986), US EPA (1986), and IARC (1989).

8.6.1 In vitro studies

In different *in vitro* assays, DMF did not induce mutations or genotoxic effects (Table 18). Negative results were obtained with both in *Salmonella typhimurium* and *Escherichia coli*. DMF did not induce unscheduled DNA synthesis, sister chromatid exchanges, chromosomal aberrations, or gene mutation in mammalian cells, or mitotic gene conversion or crossing over in yeasts (Serres & Ashby, 1981).

Table 18. Short-term genotoxicity tests on DMF (in vitro)

Method	Concentration	Condition; comment	Results	Reference
Ames test	0.65×10^{-6}-1.3×10^{-3} mol/litre	TA 98, 100, 1535, 1537, 1538, with and without liver microsome	-	Antoine et al. (1983)
B. subtilis Spore rec-assay	maximum dose 20 mg/disk	- S9, + S9 (rat, yellow tail, clam)	-	Serres & Ashby (1981)
E. coli differential killing test	highest concentration 30 µl/plate	WP2, WP67, CM871	-	Serres & Ashby (1981)
E. coli rec-assay	highest concentration 1 g/ml	2921, 9239, 8471, 5519, 7623, 7689	-	Serres & Ashby (1981)
DNA polymerase deficient assay	100 µl/ml	+ S9 and - S9 E. coli W3110 P3478	- -	Serres & Ashby (1981)
Yeast mutation		S. pombe	-	Serres & Ashby (1981)
		S. cerevisiae (XV185-14C)	-	Serres & Ashby (1981)
Mitotic recombination		S. cerevisiae (JD1)	+	Serres & Ashby (1981)
Mitotic crossing-over assay	10-1000 µg/ml	S. cerevisiae (T1, T2)	-	Serres & Ashby (1981)
Mitotic aneuploidy	lowest effective concentration 100 µg/ml	S. cerevisiae (D6) - S9	+	Serres & Ashby (1981)

Table 18 (continued)

Mitotic gene conversion	5 μl/ml	S. cerevisiae (D7) + S9	-	Serres & Ashby (1981)
Mitotic gene conversion	500 μg/ml	S. cerevisiae (JD1)	-	Serres & Ashby (1981)
Repair test using yeast strains (cell growth inhibition)	minimum effective concentration (MEC) 300 μg/ml	S. cerevisiae (wild & rad)	+	Serres & Ashby (1981)
Nuclear enlargement	0.01-100 μg/ml 8-200 μg/ml	human fibroblasts HeLa cells	- +	Serres & Ashby (1981)
UDS test	1.1-90 μg/ml (-S9) 2-30 μg/ml (+S9) 0.032-100 μg/ml 0.1-100 μg/ml	human fibroblasts (WI-38) -, + S9 human fibroblasts (from skin biopsies) HeLa cells	- - -	Serres & Ashby (1981) Serres & Ashby (1981) Serres & Ashby (1981)
Sister chromatid exchange (SCE)	0.00625-0.1% 0.1-100 μg/ml	CHO cells (-, + S9) CHO cells	- -	Serres & Ashby (1981) Serres & Ashby (1981)
RL Chromosome assay	75-300 μg/ml	Rat liver epithelial type cell line (RL1)	-	Serres & Ashby (1981)

Table 18 (continued)

Method	Concentration	Condition; comment	Results	Reference
Mouse lymphoma mutagenesis assay	46.9-3000 µg/ml	Mouse lymphoma cells (L5178Y) -, + S9 rat liver	-	Serres & Ashby (1981)
Human fibroblast Diphtheria toxin Resistance test	0.2-0.5 mg/ml	human lung fibroblast (HSC172)	-	Serres & Ashby (1981)
Cell transformation test	500 µg/ml	Baby hamster kidney cells (BHK21C13/HRC1)	+	Serres & Ashby (1981)
		BHK-21 cell	-	Serres & Ashby (1981)
Integration enhancement test (MLV Test)	0.005-0.5	C3H2K cell	-	Serres & Ashby (1981)
Cytogenetic analysis	1.1×10^{-2}-1.1 mol/litre	human peripheral lymphocytes	-	Antoine et al. (1983)
Cytogenetic analysis	10-20%	human peripheral lymphocytes	+	Koudela & Spazier (1979)

Comment: Positive results were obtained with very high concentrations, such as 100-500 µg/ml and 10-20%.

In one study, DMF did not induce any increase in chromosomal aberrations or sister chromatid exchange in human peripheral blood lymphocytes *in vitro* (Antoine et al., 1983). However, in another study, chromosomal aberrations were reported in human peripheral lymphocyte cultures treated with DMF (Koudela & Spazier, 1979). The authors performed cytogenetic analyses of human peripheral lymphocytes treated with DMF (dilution from 10^{-7} to 10^{-2} mol/litre. Compared with the positive control, thio-TEPA, the clastogenic activity of DMF was 3- to 4-fold lower. Chromosome aberrations were concentration-related at DMF levels of 10-20%.

Cytogenetic analysis of peripheral lymphocytes in 40 workers exposed to 35-180 mg DMF/m^3 was performed, first at 4-month intervals, and later at 6-month intervals. Increased frequencies of non-specified chromosomal aberrations of 3.82 and 2.74%, respectively, were found (Koudela & Spazier, 1981). In further sampling periods, after technological adjustments to decrease the DMF exposure to about 30 mg/m^3, the authors established lower frequencies of cell aberrations in most of the workers, i.e., 1.59, 1.58, and 1.49%, in the various periods under study. The aberrant cells in the control group were 1.61-1.10% (Koudela & Spazier, 1979).

8.6.2 In vivo *studies*

In *in vivo* studies, DMF was negative in dominant lethal mutagenic assays, tests for chromosome aberrations and sperm abnormalities, and micronucleus tests, (Table 19).

8.6.3 *Appraisal*

The results obtained in the *in vitro* and *in vivo* test systems showed that DMF did not induce damage in genetic material.

Table 19. Short-term genotoxicity tests of DMF (In vivo)

Method	Animal	Dose route	Results	Reference
Dominant lethal mutagenic bioassay	male rat	90, 900 mg/m^3 inhalation 6 h daily for 5 consecutive days	-	Lewis et al. (1979)
Chromosome aberrations	male and female rat	2.3-600 mg/m^3 inhalation	-	Sheveleva et al. (1979)
Micronucleus test	BALB/C mouse	0.2-2000 mg/kg ip	-	Antoine et al. (1983)
Micronucleus test	B6C3F1 mouse	80% of LD_{50} ip	-	Serres & Ashby (1981)
Micronucleus test	ICR mouse	0.425-1.7 mg/kg ip	-	Serres & Ashby (1981)
Micronucleus test	CD-1 mouse	0.4-1.6 mg/kg ip	-	Serres & Ashby (1981)
Sperm morphology assay	(CBA x BALB/c)F1 male mouse	0.1-1.5 mg/kg ip	-	Serres & Ashby (1981)

8.7 Carcinogenicity

The carcinogenic activity of DMF has not been examined in 2-year studies on test-animals (Purchase et al., 1978; Barral-Chamaillard & Rouzioux, 1983; Kennedy, 1986; US EPA, 1986). However, there are some data concerning DMF, applied as a solvent, and for shorter periods of time.

In a study by Druckrey et al. (1967) two groups of 15 and 5 BD rats were treated, with 75 and 150 mg DMF/litre in the drinking-water for 500 and 250 days, respectively (total doses 38 000 mg/litre in drinking-water). The animals were observed for up to a maximum of 750 days, with an average survival of 532 days. Similarly, two groups of 12 rats each were given weekly, subcutaneous injections of 200 and 400 mg DMF/kg (total doses 8000 and 20 000 mg/kg, respectively) and observed for 732 and 766 days, respectively. No tumorigenic effects were reported in this small group of rats.

Kommineni (1973) reported that 9 out of 18 male, and 11 out of 19 female rats, developed tumours in different organs following ip administrations of 100 mg DMF per rat, once a week, for 10 weeks. The incidence of tumours in male control rats was 4 out of 14 and, in females, 5 out of 14, also in different organs. No specific organ or tumour type predominated in either the test or control group. Three testicular tumours were seen, a bilateral interstitial cell tumour in the controls, and an interstitial cell tumour and an embryonal cell carcinoma in the test group.

8.8 Induction of tumour cell differentiation

Borenfreund et al. (1975) reported a decrease in the malignancy of the Friend erythroleukaemic cells and a marked increase in their differentiation along the erythroid pathway after their treatment with 0.5 and 1% DMF solutions.

DMF induction of cell differentiation and a marked reduction of tumorigenicity was established by Dexter (1977) in transplantable murine rhabdomyosarcoma cells. In another study, Dexter & Hager (1980) used 4 carcinoma cell lines derived from two specimens of adenosarcoma of the human sigmoid colon and showed changes in the carcinoma cells towards less malignant cell types. Hager et al.

(1980) demonstrated that a cultured human colon carcinoma cell responded to DMF by more differentiated development, again suggesting an antitumour effect.

Chakrabarty et al. (1984) studied the effects of DMF on AKR-2B and AKR-MCA cells *in vitro* and found that complete loss of anchorage independent growth occurred and the reduced expression of membrane antigens was restored.

The DMF induction of tumour cell differentiation has been studied by Kimball & Hixon (1983) in relation to the deviation of the nuclear protein. Cordeiro & Savarese (1984) studied it in relation to the effects on cysteine/glutathione metabolism, and Levine et al. (1985) in relationship to the changes in receptor occupation and growth factor responsiveness. Chen et al. (1986) studied the induction of tumour cells by DMF in relation to the rate of nucleoside transport in the cells.

A review of the studies on the effects of the induction of alkylformamides on terminal differentiation of tumour cells (Langdon & Hickman, 1987) shows that DMF should not be used for such purposes. The anti-neoplastic activity of DMF, determined *in vitro* and *in vivo*, does not appear to be sufficient for therapeutic use.

8.9 Mechanism of toxicity, mode of action

Several hypotheses on the possible mechanism of DMF hepatotoxicity have been tested. No experimental support for lipid peroxidation, lysosome labilization, or glutathione depletion has been reported. The critical biological effects leading to DMF hepatotoxicity have not been identified and still need to be elucidated (Scailteur & Lauwerys, 1987).

9. EFFECTS ON HUMAN BEINGS

9.1 General population exposure

No effects of DMF on the general population have been reported.

9.2 Occupational exposure

Reports of occupational poisonings with DMF have been reviewed by Kennedy (1986), US EPA (1986), and Scailteur & Lauwerys (1987).

9.2.1 Accidental poisoning

Several cases of acute accidental occupational poisoning with DMF have been reported (Tolot et al., 1968; Potter, 1973; Chary, 1974; Chivers, 1978; Aldyreva & Gafurov, 1980; Kang-de & Hui-lan, 1981; Shlygina & Nemolshev, 1981; Paoletti et al., 1982a,b). They were caused by the malfunctioning of the equipment, splashing of the organic solvent over the body, or working in plants without taking protective measures. Over-exposure has occurred via the skin and/or inhalation. Usually, the symptoms appeared from several hours up to several days after the accident. The major symptoms were epigastric or abdominal pain, which was irradiating and progressive, accompanied by dizziness, nausea, anorexia, vomiting, fatigue, alcohol intolerance, and skin irritation. Clinical laboratory tests showed liver function disturbance. Radioisotope diagnostic tests and liver biopsy revealed morphological changes in the liver. No clinical manifestations of renal dysfunction were reported. The patients recovered with symptomatic therapy in hospital for 2-3 weeks. Liver function tests returned to normal. Some of the patients, who were followed for several months or several years after the acute poisoning, had normal function tests.

9.2.2 Long-term exposure

After occupational exposure to DMF (intensity and length of exposure unspecified, no control groups), eye irritation, headache, anorexia, gastrointestinal disturbances, and sometimes hepatomegaly with biochemical signs of liver damage were reported. Some haematological changes were also observed (Tolot et al., 1958; Weiss, 1971; Dilorenzo & Grazioli, 1972). In studies in which exposure was quantified, subjective complaints of headache, fatigue, and gastrointestinal and cardiovascular changes were reported. Disturbances of liver function could be measured by changes in plasma bilirubin levels, and increases in the serum activity of liver enzymes (transaminases, alkaline phosphatase, glutamyl-transpeptidase). Alcohol intolerance occurred. Haematological changes and ECG deviations were also observed (Table 20).

In a questionnaire study, for which little detail is available, Schottek (1972) reported 14% miscarriages in a group of women exposed to about 100 mg DMF/m^3 compared with 10% in the control group. No statistical analysis was performed. Aldyreva & Gafurov (1980) reported perturbations in menstruation in 26 out of 70 women who had been exposed to 30-150 mg DMF/m^3 for about a year. No data are available on controls. On the basis of company statistics, general morbidity associated with gynaecological changes appeared to be increased among DMF-exposed women.

Farquharson et al. (1983) reported miscarriages in 3 out of 9 women, who had been exposed to DMF as well as a number of other chemicals.

Because of its effect on the stratum corneum, DMF interferes with the barrier function of the skin; this was demonstrated in human volunteers by increased water loss following DMF exposure (Baker, 1968).

9.2.3 *Epidemiological studies on carcinogenicity*

Ducatman et al. (1986) reported three cases of testicular germ-cell tumours in 1981-83 among 153 white men who repaired the exterior surfaces and electrical components of F4 Phantom jet aircraft, in the USA. This finding led to surveys of two other repair shops at different geographical locations; in one of the shops, the same type of aircraft was repaired, while in the other, different types of aircraft were repaired. Four out of 680 white male workers in the same type of repair shop had a history of testicular germ-cell cancers (0.95 expected) occurring in 1970-83. No case of testicular germ-cell cancer was found among the 446 white men employed at the

Table 20. Studies on workers with long-term exposures

Number of exposed subjects	Number of non-exposed controls	Length of exposure (years)	DMF exposure (mg/m³)	Urinary NMF	Hepato-toxicity	Alcohol intolerance	Other effects	Reference
22	28	5	1-47 (usually < 30; gloves worn)	20-63 mg/g creatinine	-	+	not reported	Lauwerys et al. (1980)
11	-	3	3-15	0.4-20 mg/24 h	-	+(6)[a]	not reported	Yonemoto & Suzuki (1980)
28	29	3-5	30-60	not reported	-	not reported	complaints of eye and respiratory tract irritation; no haemato-logical changes	Hinkova et al. (1980)
115	67	1-1.5	30-150 with higher peaks + skin exposure	not reported	+ (a few out of 29)	not reported	complaints of gastro-intestinal tract or cardiovascular and ovarian distur-bances (29)	Aldyreva & Gafurov (1980)
177	-	3-5	10-30	not reported	-	not reported	complaints of cardiovascular disturbances (45)	Aldyreva & Gafurov (1980)

Table 20 (continued)

Number of exposed subjects	Number of non-exposed controls	Length of exposure (years)	DMF exposure (mg/m³)	Urinary NMF	Hepato-toxicity	Alcohol intolerance	Other effects	Reference
81	96	3.5	< 10 accidental peak levels up to 4525 + skin exposure	not reported	+(10)	not reported	complaints of gastro-intestinal tract and cardiovascular disturbances, ECG changes	Kang-de & Hui-Lan (1981)
23	-	2	> 30 peaks up to 150	10-40 mg/day	not reported	not reported	No ECG changes compared with pre-exposure	Taccola et al. (1981)
27	237	2	2-80 peaks up to 549	not reported	+(2)	+(8)	complaints of gastro-intestinal tract disturbances (15); headache (6)	Paoletti & Iannaccone (1982)
13	-	≤ 4	14-60 (mean: 29)	not reported	+(2)	+(8)	complaints of gastro-intestinal tract disturbances (8); eye irritation (11); kidney function test and haematology, normal	Tomasini et al (1983)

Table 20 (continued)

26	54	> 5	2-5 (mean: 3)	not reported	-	not reported	not reported	Catenacci et al. (1984)
28	54	> 5	12-25 (mean: 18)	not reported	-	not reported	not reported	Catenacci et al. (1984)
100	100	5	8-58 (mean: 22)	not reported	+ (8 versus 2 controls)	+ (39)	complaints of headache, eye and throat irritation, gastro-intestinal tract and cardiovascular disturbance	Cirla et al. (1984)
24	29	5	10-60	not reported	not reported	not reported	irritative dermatitis	Bainova (1985)
15	28	6-10	20-30 (median 27)	not reported	not reported	not reported	increased coagulation time	Imbriani et al. (1986)

a Incidence is indicated when available.

facility where different types of aircraft were repaired. Of the 7 cases of testicular germ cell tumours, 5 were seminomas and 2 were embryonal-cell carcinomas. All 7 men had long histories of working in aircraft repair. The time from first exposure to diagnosis ranged from 4 to 19 years. There were many common exposures to solvents in the three facilities, the only exposure identified as unique to the F4 Phantom jet aircraft repair facilities, where the cases occurred, being to a solvent mixture containing 80% dimethylformamide (20% unspecified). No quantitative exposure data exist. Three of the cases had certainly been exposed to this mixture and 3 cases, probably exposed. The cases were found through foremen and from filed death certificates, and the authors suggested that underreporting was possible. No other cases of cancer were investigated.

Levin et al. (1987) described 3 cases of embryonal-cell carcinoma of the testes in workers at one leather tannery in the USA, all of whom had worked as swabbers on the spray lines in leather finishing. The latency period was from 8 to 14 years. According to the authors, all the tanneries surveyed used dimethylformamide, as well as a wide range of dyes, solvents, and other chemicals. No quantitative exposure data are available. The number of workers from which these 3 cases arose was not given, and other cancers were not looked for.

To evaluate the significance of this cluster, an analysis of the New York State Cancer Registry was conducted. Occupations were determined from cancer registries and from death certificates for all residents in Fulton County who were diagnosed as having testicular cancer from 1974-88. From preliminary results, it is estimated that workers who are employed in the leather tanning industry are 5-6 times more likely to develop testicular cancer than those who are not leather workers. However, the testicular cancer rates in this county were lower than expected within this period, and an adjacent county showed the same number of cases of testicular cancer, none of the affected individuals having ever worked in the leather industry (Walrath et al., 1988).

O'Berg et al. (1985) and Chen et al. (1988a) studied the cancer incidence among 2530 actively employed workers with potential exposure to dimethylformamide between 1956 and 1984, 1329 employees with exposure to dimethylformamide and acrylonitrile at an acrylic fibre manufacturing plant in South Carolina, USA, and 1130 controls from the same plant. Cancer incidence rates for the company (1956-84) and USA national rates (1973-77) were used to calculate the expected number of cases. For all workers exposed to DMF (alone or with acrylonitrile), the standardized incidence ratio (SIR), based on company rates for all cancers combined, was 110 [95% confidence interval (CI), 88-136]* (88 cases); the SIR on the basis of national rates was 92. The SIR for cancer of the buccal cavity and pharynx was 344 [CI, 172-615]* (11 cases), on the basis of company rates, and 167, on the basis of US rates. More cancer cases than expected from company rates (34 cases: SIR 134 [CI, 98-195]*) were found among employees exposed to dimethylformamide alone, due mainly to 8 carcinomas of the buccal cavity and pharynx versus 1.0 expected (SIR, 800 [CI, 345-1580]*). All of these cases either smoked or chewed tobacco, but no information was available on the smoking, tobacco chewing, or drinking habits of the cohort. An additional case occurred among employees exposed to dimethylformamide alone (SIR, 167); 4 of these tumours were cancers of the lip. No such excess was found among the workers exposed to both dimethylformamide and acrylonitrile (2 observed; SIR, 125, on the basis of company rates). The authors reported that there was no association with intensity or duration of exposure: "low" and "moderate" exposure SIR 420 (5 cases); "high" exposure SIR 300 (6 cases). "Low" exposure conditions included: no direct contact with liquids containing any dimethylformamide, even wearing protective equipment; and workplace air levels consistently below 30 mg DMF/m^3 (10 ppm) (no odour of DMF evident). "Moderate" exposure conditions included: intermittent contact with liquids containing > 5% dimethylformamide; workplace air levels sometimes higher than 30 mg DMF/m^3 (10 ppm) (more than once per week); DMF-laden materials handled, but air levels of DMF maintained at above levels. "High" exposure conditions included: frequent contact with liquids containing > 5% dimethylformamide; workplace air levels often > 30 mg DMF/m^3 (> 10 ppm); use of breathing protection often required for periods of 15 min-1 h; DMF vapour levels frequently > 30 mg/m^3 (> 10 ppm) (when handling

---

* As calculated by IARC (1989).

Effects on human beings

pure dimethylformamide or dimethylformamide-containing materials). One case of testicular cancer was found among the 3859 workers exposed to DMF (alone or with acrylonitrile) with 1.7 expected on the basis of company rates, and no cases of liver cancer. The company rates may be more relevant for comparison, as there were only actively employed persons among the exposed and because the USA rates are based on a limited time period, 1973-77.

Chen et al. (1988b) analysed mortality from 1950-82 among both active and pensioned employees in the same cohort. Expected numbers (adjusted for age and time period) were based on company rates. For all workers exposed to DMF (alone or with acrylonitrile), the standardized mortality ratio (SMR) for lung cancer was 124 (33 cases [95% CI, 85-174]^a). An increased risk of lung cancer was found in the cohort exposed only to DMF (19 cases; SMR 141 [CI, 84-219]^a), but not in the cohort exposed to DMF and acrylonitrile. There were 3 deaths from cancer of the buccal cavity and pharynx (SIR 188) in all persons exposed to DMF (alone or with acrylonitrile). No other excess cancer risk was reported. No information is given in this report on loss to follow-up, death certificates, or whether these deaths were included in the incidence study reported above.

Walrath et al. (1988) reported a case-control study on cancer among 8724 Du Pont employees with potential exposure to DMF in 4 other USA plants. Summary analyses for all plants combined did not show any statistically significant association between ever having been exposed to DMF and subsequent development of cancers of the buccal cavity and pharynx, liver, malignant melanoma, prostate, and testes. When odds ratios are examined according to plant site, prostate cancer at one site was significantly elevated, on the basis of 3 cases exposed out of 4, but no statistically significant association was observed among employees similarly exposed to DMF in the other 3 plants. The recency of exposure to DMF, the low exposures received, and the absence of similar excesses at other plants argue against a causal association between DMF exposure and prostate cancer at the one site. Assessment of highest DMF exposure rank,

---

^{a} As calculated by IARC (1989).

duration of exposure, and latent period, does not show any patterns suggesting an association between DMF and cancers of the buccal cavity and pharynx, liver, malignant melanoma, prostate, or testes.

9.2.4 Alcohol intolerance

Reviews on the synergistic action of ethanol with organic solvents have been published by Haguenoer et al. (1982), Hills & Venable (1982), and Stockley (1983).

Episodes of alcohol intolerance among workers exposed to DMF have been repeatedly described at all levels of exposure (see sections 9.2.1 and 9.2.2, and Table 20).

Symptoms include flushing of the face, dizziness, nausea, tightness of the chest, sometimes dyspnoea, and cardiac palpitations. The reactions were reported within 24 h of DMF exposure and very shortly after alcohol ingestion. These episodes lasted for up to 2 h (Chivers, 1978; Lyle et al., 1979; Yonemoto & Suzuki, 1980; Paoletti et al., 1982a; Cirla et al., 1984).

According to Loos (1979), abnormal liver function tests were already discovered among workers who drank only 50-70 g alcohol per day, but were also exposed to 45-66 mg DMF/m^3, while the threshold consumption for functional liver changes was 80-100 g alcohol per day in control individuals. It should be noted that the test group was also exposed to other solvents, mainly tetrahydrofuran, toluene, and xylene.

10. PREVIOUS EVALUATIONS BY INTERNATIONAL BODIES

The International Agency for Research on Cancer (IARC) evaluated the carcinogenicity of dimethylformamide in 1988 (IARC, 1989), and concluded that:

- there is *limited evidence* for the carcinogenicity of dimethylformamide in humans;
- there is *inadequate evidence* for the carcinogenicity of dimethylformamide in experimental animals.

Overall evaluation: Dimethylformamide is possibly carcinogenic to humans (Group 2B).

REFERENCES

ALDYREVA, M.V. & GAFUROV, S.A. (1980) [*Labour protection in the production of artificial leather.*] Moscow, Medizina, 158 pp (in Russian).

ALDYREVA, M.V., BORTSEVICH, S.V., PALAGUSHINA, A.I., SIDOROVA, N.V., & TARASOVA, L.A. (1980) [Effect of dimethylformamide on workers' health in the production of polyurethane synthetic leather.] *Gig. Tr. prof. Zabol.*, **6**: 24-28 (in Russian).

AMSTER, M.B., HIJAZI, N., & CHAN, R. (1983) Real time monitoring of low level air contaminants from hazardous waste sites. In: *Proceedings of the National Conference on Management of Uncontrolled Hazardous Waste Sites. Washington, DC*, pp. 98-99.

ANTOINE, J.L., ARANY, J., LEONARD, A., HENROTTE, J., JENAR-DUBUISSON, G., & DECAT, G. (1983) Lack of mutagenic activity of dimethylformamide. *Toxicology*, **26**: 207-212.

ARENA, N., SANTA CRUZ, G., ALIA, E.F., BALDUS, M., CORGIOLU, T., & ALIA, E.E. (1982) [Structural and ultrastructural changes in the myocardium of rabbits exposed to dimethylformamide vapours.] *Boll. Soc. Ital. Biol. Sper.*, **58**: 1496-1501 (in Italian).

BAINOVA, A. (1980) [Contemporary views on the hygiene standardization of dimethylformamide.] *Letopisi HEI*, **37**: 62-68 (in Bulgarian).

BAINOVA, A. (1985) [*Toxicological problems due to the action of chemical substances on the skin (dermatotoxicology).*] Sofia, Referat, pp. 1-60 (D. Sci. Thesis) (in Bulgarian).

BAINOVA, A. & ANTOV, G. (1980) Dermal toxicity of dimethylformamide in rats. In: *Abstracts of the 5th International Symposium on Occupational Health in the Production of Artificial Fibres, Belgirate, Italy, 16-20 September, 1980,* Modena, Permanent Commission and International Association on Occupational Health, pp. 73-74.

BAINOVA, A., SPASSOVSKI, M., HINKOVA, L., & TASHEVA, M. (1981a) [Effect of intermittent and continuous action of dimethylformamide on the adaptation process.] *Probl. hig.*, **6**: 27-35 (in Bulgarian).

BAINOVA, A., ANTOV, G.P., & IVANOVICH, E.H. (1981b) Combined action of dimethylformamide and noise on kidneys of white rats. *CR. Acad. bulg. Sci.*, **34**: 1609-1611.

BAKER, H. (1968) The effects of dimethylsulfoxide, dimethylformamide, and dimethylacetamide on the cutaneous barrier to water in human skin. *J. invest. Dermatol.*, **50**: 283-288.

BARNES, J.R. & HENRY, N.W. (1974) The determination of N-methylformamide and N-methylacetamide in urine. *Am. Ind. Hyg. Assoc. J.*, **35**: 84-87.

BARNES, J.R. & RANTA, K.E. (1972) The metabolism of dimethylformamide and dimethylacetamide. *Toxicol. appl. Pharmacol.*, **23**: 271-276.

BARRAL-CHAMAILLARD, J. & ROUZIOUX, M. (1983) Dimethylformamide. *Arch. Mal. prof.*, **44**: 203-208.

BARTSCH, W., SPONER, G., DIETMAN, K., & FUCHS, G. (1976) Acute toxicity of various solvents in the mouse and rat. *Arzneimittelforschung*, **26**: 1581-1583.

BECCI, P.J., VOSS, K.A., JOHNSON, W.D., GALLO, M.A., & BABISH, J.G. (1983) Subchronic feeding study of N,N-dimethylformamide in rats and mice. *J. Am. Coll. Toxicol.*, **2**(6): 371-378.

BEGERT, A. (1975) [Purification of chemical textile plant sewage.] *Oesterr. Abwasser-Rundsch.*, **20**: 98-102 (in German).

BORENFREUND, E., STEINGLASS, M., KORNGOLD, G., & BENDICH, A. (1975) Effect of dimethylsulfoxide and dimethylformamide on the growth and morphology of tumour cells. *Ann. N.Y. Acad. Sci.*, **243**: 164-171.

BORTSEVICH, S.V. (1984) [The hygienic importance of dimethylformamide absorption through the skin.] *Gig. Tr. prof. Zabol.*, **11**: 55-57 (in Russian).

BRINDLEY, C., GESCHER, A., & ROSS, D. (1983) Studies of the metabolism of dimethylformamide in mice. *Chem.-biol. Interact.*, **45**: 387-392.

BRONDEAU, M.T., BONNET, P., GUENIER, J.P., & DE CEAURRIZ, J. (1983) Short-term inhalation test for evaluating industrial hepatotoxicants in rats. *Toxicol. Lett.*, **19**: 139-146.

BRUGNONE, F., PERBELLINI, L., & GAFFURI, E. (1980a) N,N-Dimethylformamide concentration in environmental and alveolar air in a artificial leather factory. *Br. J. ind. Med.*, **37**: 185-188.

BRUGNONE, F., PERBELLINI, L., GAFFURI, E., & ASASTOLI, P. (1980b) Biomonitoring of industrial solvent exposures in workers' alveolar air. *Int. Arch. occup. environ. Health*, **47**: 245-261.

BRUGNONE, F., PERBELLINI, L., GAFFURI, E., & TURRI, P.V. (1984) Monitoring of industrial exposure to dimethylformamide by analysis of alveolar air. *Med. Lav.*, **6**: 139-141.

BURGUN, J., MARTZ, R., FORNEY, R.B., & KIPLINGER, G.F. (1975) The acute toxicity of dimethylformamide and its combined effects with ethanol in the mouse. *Toxicol. appl. Pharmacol.*, **33**: 149-150.

References

CAI, S.X. & HUANG, M.Y. (1979) Investigation on occupational hazard in a butadiene monomer workshop of a *cis*-butadiene rubber plant. *J. Hyg. Res.*, **8**(1): 22-49 (in Chinese).

CARDWELL, R.D., FOREMAN, D.G., PAYNE, T.R., & WILBUR, D.J. (1978) *Acute and chronic toxicity of four chemicals to fish*. Duluth, Minnesota, US Environmental Protection Agency (Contract 68-01-0711).

CATENACCI, G., GRAMPELLA, D., TERZI, R., SALA, H., & POLLINI, G., (1984) Hepatic function in subjects exposed to environmental concentrations of DMF lower than the actually proposed TLV. *Med. Lav.*, **6**: 157-158.

CHAKRABARTY, S., MCRAE, L.J., LEVINE, A.E., & BRATTAIX, M.G. (1984) Restoration of normal growth control and membrane antigen composition in malignant cells by *N,N*-dimethylformamide. *Cancer Res.*, **44**: 2181-2185.

CHARY, S. (1974) Dimethylformamide. A case of acute pancreatitis. *Lancet*, **2**(7876): 356.

CHEN, J.L., FAYERWEATHER, W.E., & PELL, S. (1988a) Cancer incidence of workers exposed to dimethylformamide and/or acrylonitrile. *J. occup. Med.*, **30**: 813-818.

CHEN, J.L., FAYERWEATHER, W.E., & PELL, S. (1988b) Mortality study of workers exposed to dimethylformamide and/or acrylonitrile. *J. occup. Med.*, **30**: 819-821.

CHEN, S.-F., CLEAVELAND, J.S., HOLLMAN, A.B., WIEMANN, M.C., PARKS, R.E., & STOECKLER, J.D. (1986) Changes in nucleoside transport of HL-60 human promyelocytic cells during *N,N*-dimethylformamide induced differentiation. *Cancer Res.*, **46**: 3449-3455.

CHIVERS, C.P. (1978) Disulfiram effect from inhalation of dimethylformamide. *Lancet*, **1**(8059): 331.

CHROMEK, J., KUPEK, J., MLADEK, M., & MARVAN, P. (1983) A study of respiration of the alga *Sceadesmus quadricauda* in batch conditions under influence of *N,N*-dimethylformamide and dimethylamine. *Arch. Hydrobiol.*, **64**(Suppl.): 441-460.

CIRLA, A.M., PISATI, G., INVERNIZZI, E., & TORRICELLI, P. (1984) Epidemiological study on workers exposed to low dimethylformamide concentrations. *G. Ital. Med. Lav.*, **6**: 149-156.

CLAY, P.F. & SPITTLER, T.M. (1983) Determination of airborne volatile nitrogen compounds using four independent techniques. In: *Proceedings of the National Conference on Management of Uncontrolled Hazardous Waste Sites, Washington, DC*, pp. 100-104.

CLAYTON, J.W., BARNES, J.R., HOOD, D.B., & SCHEPERS, G.W. (1963) The inhalation toxicity of dimethylformamide (DMF). *Am. Ind. Hyg. Assoc. J.*, **24**: 144-154.

CORDEIRO, R.F. & SAVARESE, T.M. (1984) Reversal by L-cysteine of the growth inhibitory and glutathione-depleting effects of N-methylformamide and N,N-dimethylformamide. *Biochem. biophys. Res. Commun.*, **122**: 798-803.

COSTA, V., FRONGIA, N., & SANTA CRUZ, G. (1978) [Histological and ultrastructural changes of the rat renal glomerulus caused by dimethylformamide inhalation.] *Boll. Soc. Ital. Biol. Sper.*, **54**: 1723-1728 (in Italian).

CRAIG, D.K., WEIR, R.J., WAGNER, W., & GROTH, D. (1984) Subchronic inhalation toxicity of dimethylformamide in rats and mice. *Drug chem. Toxicol.*, **7**: 551-571.

DARNALL, K.R., LLOYD, A.C., WINER, A.M., & PITTS, J.N. (1976) Reactivity scale for atmospheric hydrocarbons based on reaction with hydroxyl radical. *Environ. Sci. Technol.*, **7**: 692-696.

DEXTER, D.L. (1977) N,N-Dimethylformamide-induced morphological differentiation and reduction of tumorigenicity in cultured mouse rhabdomyosarcoma cells. *Cancer Res.*, **37**: 3136-3140.

DEXTER, D.L. & HAGER, J.C. (1980) Maturation induction of tumour cells using a human colon carcinoma model. *Cancer*, **45**: 1178-1184.

DILORENZO, F. & GRAZIOLI, C. (1972) [Hematological, hematochemical, and gastric findings in workers exposed to breathing vapours of dimethylformamide.] *Lav. Um.*, **24**: 96-106 (in Italian).

DIXON, S.W., GRAEPEL, G.J., & LOONEY, W.C. (1983) Seasonal effects on concentrations of monomethylformamide in urine samples. *Am. Ind. Hyg. Assoc. J.*, **44**: 273-275.

DOJLIDO, J.R. (1979) *Investigations of biodegradability and toxicity of organic compounds.* Washington, DC, US Environmental Protection Agency (Unpublished report No. EPA-600/2-79-163).

DRUCKREY, H., PREUSSMANN, R., IVANKOVIC, S., & SCHMAHL, D. (1967) [Organotropic carcinogenic effects of 65 different N-nitroso-compounds on B.D. rats.] *Z. Krebsforsch.*, **69**: 103-201 (in German).

DUCATMAN, A.M., CONWILL, D.E., & CRAWL, J. (1986) Germ cell tumours of the testicle among aircraft repairmen. *J. Urol.*, **136**: 834-836.

EBEN, A. & KIMMERLE, G. (1976) Metabolism studies in N,N-dimethylformamide. III. Studies on the influence of ethanol in persons and laboratory animals. *Int. Arch. occup. environ. Health*, **36**: 243-265.

References

EBERLING, C.L. (1980) Formic acid and derivatives (DMF). In: *Kirk-Othmer encyclopedia of chemical technology*, 3rd ed., New York, Chichester, Brisbane, Toronto, John Wiley & Sons, Vol. 11, pp. 263-268.

ELOVAARA, E., MARSELOS, M., & VAINO, H. (1983) N,N-Dimethylformamide-induced effects on hepatic and renal xenobiotic enzymes with emphasis on aldehyde metabolism in the rat. *Acta. pharmacol. toxicol.*, **53**: 159-165.

EWING, B.B., CHIAN, E.S.K., COOK, J.C., EVANS, C.A., HOPKE, P.A., & PERKINS, E.G. (1977) *Monitoring to detect previously unrecognized pollutants in surface water. Appendix: Organic analysis data*, Washington, DC, US Environmental Protection Agency, (Unpublished report No. EPA-560/6-77-015).

FARHI, M., MOREL, M., & CAVIGNEAUX, A. (1968) Dimethylformamide. $NCON(CH_3)_2$. *Cah. Notes doc.*, **50**: 91-93.

FARLEY, F.F. (1977) Photochemical reactivity classification of hydrocarbons and other organic compounds. In: *International Conference on Photochemical Oxidant Pollution and Its Containment*, Research Triangle Park, North Carolina, US Environmental Protection Agency. (Unpublished report No. EPA-600/3-77-0018).

FARQUHARSON, R.O., HALL, M.A., & FULLERTON, W.T. (1983) Poor obstetric outcome in three quality control laboratory workers. *Lancet*, **30**: 983-984.

GERMANOVA, A.L., HALEPO, A.I., AVILOVA, G.G., ANVAER, L., HOROCHULOVA, N.V., MALTSEVA, N.M., & MIGUKINA, N.V. (1979) [Adaptation after continuous and intermittent exposure to dimethylformamide.] In: *[The toxicology of new industrial chemicals.]* Moscow, Medizina, Vol. 15, pp. 69-76 (in Russian).

GRASSELLI, J.G. (1973) *Atlas of spectral data and physical constants for organic compounds*, Cleveland, Ohio, USA, The Chemical Rubber Co.

GUBSER, H. (1969) Purification of chemical waste waters. *Gas Wasser Abwasser*, **49**: 175-181.

HAGER, J.C., GOLD, D.V., BARBOSA, J.A., FLIGIEL, L., MILLER, F., & DEXTER, D.L. (1980) N,N-Dimethylformamide-induced modulation of organ and tumour associated markers in cultured human colon carcinoma cells. *J. Natl Cancer Inst.*, **64**: 439-445.

HAGUENOER, J.M., BOURRINET, P., & FRIMAT, P. (1982) Interrelations between alcoholism and exposure to industrial poisons. *Arch. Mal. prof.*, **43**: 461-473.

HAMILTON, A. & HARDY, H.L. (1974) *Industrial toxicology*, 3rd ed., Acton, Massachusetts, Publishing Science Group Inc., 349 pp.

HANASONO, G.K., FULLER, R.W., BRODDLE, W.D., & GIBSON, W.R. (1977) Studies on the effects of N,N-dimethylformamide on ethanol disposition and on monoamine oxidase activity in rats. *Toxicol. appl. Pharmacol.*, **39**: 461-472.

HELLWIG, J., MERKLE, J., KLIMISCH, H.J., & JACKH, R. (in press) Investigations on the prenatal toxicity of N,N-dimethylformamide (DMF) in mice, rats and rabbits. *Food chem. Toxicol.*.

HENRY, N.W. & SCHLATTER, C.N. (1981) The development of a standard method for evaluating chemical protective clothing to permeation by hazardous liquids. *Am. Ind. Hyg. Assoc. J.*, **42**: 202-207.

HILLS, B.W. & VENABLE (1982) The interaction of ethyl alcohol and industrial chemicals. *Am. J. ind. Med.*, **3**: 321-333.

HINKOVA, L., GINCHEVA, N., STAMOVA, N., HRISTEVA, V., CHOLAKOV, B., & SASSOVSKY, M. (1980) [Influence of dimethylformamide on workers' health.] *Probl. hyg., Sofia*, **5**: 75-81 (in Bulgarian).

HUANG, M.Y., LUO, Y.Z., GENG, T.B., MENG, D.S., LIU, J., HUANG, M.F., & WANG, Y.S. (1981) [Studies on the dermal toxicity of dimethylformamide.] *J. Hyg. Res.*, **10**(4): 21-26 (in Chinese).

HUGHES, J.S. & VILKAS A.G. (1983) Toxicity of N,N-dimethylformamide used as a solvent in toxicity tests with the green alga *Selenastrum capricornum*. *Bull. environ. Contam. Toxicol.*, **31**: 98-104.

IARC (1989) Dimethylformamide. In: *Some organic solvents, resin monomers and related compounds, pigments and occupational exposures in paint manufacture and painting*, Lyon, International Agency for Research on Cancer, pp. 171-197 (IARC Monograph on the Evaluation of Carcinogenic Risks to Humans, Vol. 47).

IMBRIANI, M., CHITTORI, S., PRESTINONI, A., LONGONI, P., CASCONE, G., & GAMBA, G. (1986) Effects of dimethylformamide (DMF) on coagulation and platelet activity. *Arch. environ. Health*, **41**: 90-93.

KANG-DE, C. & HUI-LAN, Z. (1981) Observation on the effects of dimethylformamide on human health. In: *Abstracts of the 9th International Congress on Occupational Health in the Chemical Industry, Aswan, Egypt, 15-17 September 1981*, Aswan, Egypt, Permanent Commission and International Association on Occupational Health, pp. 22-23.

KELLER, C.A. & LEWIS, S.C. (1981) Inhalation teratology study of N,N-dimethylformamide (DMF). *Teratology*, **23**: 45A.

References

KENNEDY, G.L., Jr (1986) Biological effects of acetamide, formamide, and their monomethyl and dimethyl derivatives. *CRC crit. Rev. Toxicol.*, **17**(2), 129-182.

KENNEDY, G.L. & SHERMAN, H. (1986) Acute and subchronic toxicity of dimethylformamide and dimethylacetamide following various routes of administration. *Drug chem. Toxicol.*, **9**: 147-170.

KESTELL, P., GILL, M.H., THREADGILL, M.D., GESCHER, A., HOWARTH, O.W., & CURZON, E.H. (1986) Identification by proton NMR of N-(hydroxymethyl)-N-methylformamide as the major urinary metabolite of N,N-dimethylformamide in mice. *Life Sci.*, **38**: 719-724.

KESTELL, P., THREADGILL, M.D., GESCHER, A., GLEDHILL, A.P., SHAW, A.J., & FARMER, R.B. (1987) An investigation of the relationship between the hepatotoxicity and the metabolism of N-alkylformamides. *J. Pharmacol. exp. Ther.*, **270**: 265-270.

KIMBALL, P.M. & HIXON, S. (1983) Nuclear protein changes following N,N-dimethylformamide (DMF) induced maturation. *J. cell. Biochem.*, **22**: 245-249.

KIMMERLE, G. & EBEN, A. (1975a) Metabolism studies of N,N-dimethylformamide. I. Studies in rats and dogs. *Int. Arch. Arbeitsmed.*, **34**: 109-126.

KIMMERLE, G. & EBEN, A. (1975b) Metabolism studies of N,N-dimethylformamide. II. Studies in persons. *Int. Arch. Arbeitsmed.*, **34**: 127-136.

KIMMERLE, G. & MACHEMER, L. (1975) Studies with N,N-dimethylformamide for embryotoxic and teratogenic effects on rats after dynamic inhalation. *Int. Arch. Arbeitsmed.*, **34**: 167-175.

KIMURA, E.T., EBERT, D.M., & DODGE, P.W. (1971) Acute toxicity and limits of solvent residue for sixteen organic solvents. *Toxicol. appl. Pharmacol.*, **19**(4): 699-704.

KISS, G. (1979) [Study of the irritative action of dimethylformamide.] *Börg. Venerol.*, **55**: 203 (in Hungarian).

KOMMINENI, C. (1973) *Pathological studies of aflatoxin fractions and dimethylformamide in MRC rats*, Omaha, University of Nebraska (Dissertation, December 1972).

KOUDELA, K. & SPAZIER, K. (1979) [Effects of dimethylformamide on human peripheral lymphocytes.] *Cesk. Hyg.*, **24**: 432-436 (in Czech).

KOUDELA, K. & SPAZIER, K. (1981) [Increased concentration of dimethylformamide vapours in the atmosphere.] *Prac. Lek.*, **33**: 121-123 (in Czech).

KRAMER, V.C., SCHNELL, D.J., & NICKERSON, K.W. (1983) Relative toxicity of organic solvents to *Aedes aegypti* larvae. *J. invertebr. Pathol.*, **42**: 285-287.

KRIVANEK, N.D., MCLAUGHLIN, M., & FAYERWEATHER, W.E. (1978) Monomethylformamide levels in human urine after repetitive exposure to dimethylformamide vapour. *J. occup. Med.*, **20**: 179-182.

LAITY, J.L., BURSTEIN, I.G., & APPEL, B.R. (1973) Photochemical smog and the atmospheric reactions of solvents. In: *Solvents theory and practice*, pp. 95-112, Washington, DC, American Chemical Society (Advances in Chemistry Series, Vol. 124).

LANGDON, S.P. & HICKMAN, J.A. (1987) Alkylformamides as inducers of tumour cell differentiation - a mini-review. *Toxicology*, **43**: 239-249.

LAUWERYS, R. (1986) Dimethylformamide. In: Alessio, L., Berlin, A., Boni, M., & Roi, R., ed. *Biological indicators for the assessment of human exposure to industrial chemicals.* Brussels, Luxembourg, Commission of the European Communities Joint Research Centre, pp. 19-27.

LAUWERYS, R.R., KIVITS, A., LHOIR, M., RIGOLET, P., HOUBAT, D., BUCHET, J.P., & ROELS, H.A. (1980) Biological surveillance of workers exposed to dimethylformamide and the influence of skin protection on its percutaneous absorption. *Int. Arch. occup. environ. Health*, **45**: 189-203.

LAZAREV, N.V. & LEVINA, E.N. (1976) [Dimethylformamide.] In: [Harmful substances in industry.] Leningrad, Khimia, Vol. 2, pp. 36-38 (in Russian).

LEBLANC, G.A. & SURPRENANT, D.C. (1983) The acute and chronic toxicity of acetone, dimethylformamide, and triethylene glycol to *Daphnia magna* (Strauss). *Arch. environ. Contam. Toxicol.*, **12**: 305-310.

LESHIK, J.A.D. & FEOKTISTOVA, A.J. (1984) [Ascorbic acid supply and cytochrome P-450 level in guinea-pig liver during dimethylformamide poisoning.] *J. Vopr. Pitan.*, **5**: 65-67 (in Russian).

LEVIN, S.M., BAKER, D.B., LANDRIGAN, P.J., MONAGHAN, S.V., FRUMIN, E., BRAITHWAITE, M., & TOWNE, W. (1987) Testicular cancer in leather tanners exposed to dimethylformamide. *Lancet*, **II**(8568): 1153.

LEVINE, A.E., MCRAE, L.J., & BRATTAIN, M.G. (1985) Changes in receptor occupancy and growth factor responsiveness induced by treatment of a transformed mouse embryo cell line with N,N-dimethylformamide. *Cancer Res.*, **45**: 6401-6405.

LEWIS, S.C., RINEHART, W.E., SCHROEDER, R.E., & THAKARA, J.W. (1979) Dominant lethal mutagenic bioassay of dimethylformamide (DMF). *Environ. Mutagen.*, **1**: 166.

References

LIPSKI, K. (1982) Liquid chromatographic determinations of dimethylformamide, methylene bisphenyl isocyanate, and methylene bisphenyl amine in air samples. *Ann. occup. Hyg.*, **25**: 1-4.

LLEWELLYN, G.C., HASTINGS, W.C., & KIMBROUGH, T.D. (1974) The effects of dimethylformamide on female Mongolian gerbils *Meriones unguiculatus*. *Bull. environ. Contam. Toxicol.*, **11**: 467-473.

LOBANOVA, K.P. (1958) [Toxicity of dimethylformamide.] *Gig. i Sanit.*, **23**: 31-37 (in Russian).

LOOS, H. (1979) Hazards, health supervision, and potentiation of alcohol by mixtures of organic solvents, especially dimethylformamide (DMF). *Arbeitsmed. Sozialmed. Präventivmed.*, **14**(5): 127-129.

LUNDBERG, I., LUNDBERG, S., & KRONEVY, T. (1981) Some observations on dimethylformamide hepatotoxicity. *Toxicology*, **22**: 1-7.

LUNDBERG, I., PEHRSSON, A., LUNDBERG, S., KRONEVY, T., & LIDUMS, V. (1983) Delayed dimethyformamide biotransformation after high exposures in rats. *Toxicol. Lett.*, **17**: 29-34.

LUNDBERG, I., EKDAHL, M., KRONEVI, T., LIDUMS, V., & LUNDBERG, S. (1986) Relative hepatotoxicity of some industrial solvents after intraperitoneal injection or inhalation exposure in rats. *Environ. Res.*, **40**: 411-420.

LUNDBERG, S. (1982) [*Nordic group of experts for documentation of threshold limit values - 38. Dimethylformamide.*] Solna, Sweden, National Institute of Occupational Health, pp. 32 (Report 1982:28) (in Swedish).

LYLE, W.H., SPENCE, T.W.M., MCKINNELEY, W.M., & DUCKERS, K. (1979) Dimethylformamide and alcohol intolerance. *Br. J. ind. Med.*, **36**: 63-66.

MALONOVA, H. & BARDODEJ, Z. (1983) Urinary excretion of mercapturates as a biological indicator of exposure to electrophilic agents. *J. Hyg. epidem. Microbiol. Immunol.*, **27**(3): 319-328.

MASSMANN, W. (1956) Toxicological investigations on dimethylformamide. *Br. J. ind. Med.*, **13**: 51-54.

MATHEW, T., KARUNANITHY, R., YEE, M.H., & NATARAJAN, P.N. (1980) Hepatotoxicity of dimethylformamide and dimethylsulfoxide at and above the levels used in some aflatoxin studies. *Lab. Invest.*, **42**: 257-262.

MAXFIELD, M.E., BARNES, J.R., AZAR, A., & TROCHIMOWIEZ, H.T. (1975) Urinary excretion of metabolite following experimental human exposure to dimethylformamide or to dimethylacetamide. *J. occup. Med.*, **17**: 506-511.

MEDYANKIN, A.V. (1975) [Complex action of dimethylformamide under conditions of a long-term experiment.] *Gig. i Sanit.*, **9**: 39-42 (in Russian).

MERKLE, J. VON. & ZELLER, H. (1980) [Studies on acetamides and formamides for embryotoxic and teratogenic activities in the rabbit.] *Arzneimittelforschung*, **30**: 1557-1562 (in German).

MRAZ, J. & TURECEK, F. (1987) Identification of N-acetyl-S-(N-methylcarbamoyl) cysteine, a human metabolite of N',N'-dimethylformamide and N-methylformamide. *J. Chromatogr.*, **414**: 399-404.

MRAZ, J., MRAZ, M., SEDIVEC, V., & FLEK, J. (1987) [Gas chromatographic determination of N-methylformamide in urine.] *Pra. Lek.*, **39**: 352-355 (in Czech).

MURAVIEVA, S.I. (1983) [Improvement of the methods for monitoring the content of harmful substances in the air of worksite.] *Gig. Tr. prof. Zabol.*, **6**: 39-41 (in Russian).

MURAVIEVA, S.I. & ANVAER, L.P. (1979) [Determination of dimethylformamide and its metabolites in biological liquids by gas chromatographic method.] *Gig. Tr. prof. Zabol.*, **6**: 58-59 (in Russian).

O'BERG, M.T., CHEN, J.L., & BURKE, C.A. (1985) Epidemiologic study of workers exposed to acrylonitrile, an update. *J. occup. Med.*, **27**: 835-840.

ODOSHASHVILI, D.G. (1963) [Hygienic evaluation of atmospheric air pollution with dimethylformamide.] In: [Literature on air pollution and related occupational diseases.] Vol. 9, pp. 169-177 (in Russian).

PAOLETTI, A. & IANNACCONE, A. (1982) [Risk from dimethylformamide intoxication in a plant for synthetic leather.] *Ann. Ist. Super. Sanit.*, **18**: 567-570 (in Italian).

PAOLETTI, A., FABRI, G., & MASCI, O. (1982a) [Antabuse effect from solvents: comparison between dimethylformamide and trichloroethylene.] *Ann. Ist. Super. Sanit.*, **14**: 1099-1100 (in Italian).

PAOLETTI, A., FABRI, G., & MARINI BETTOLO, P. (1982b) [An isolated case of "acute abdomen". Intoxication from dimethylformamide.] *Minerva Med.*, **73**: 3407-3410 (in Italian).

PARKHIE, M. & WEBB, M. (1983) Embryotoxicity and teratogenicity of thalidomide in rats. *Teratology*, **27**: 327.

References

PERRY, D.L., CHUANG, C.C., JUNGCLAUS, G.A., & WARNER, J.S. (1979) *Identification of organic compounds in industrial effluent discharges*, Athens, Georgia, US Environmental Protection Agency, Office of Research and Development (Unpublished report No. EPA-600/4-79-016, NTIS PB-294794).

PHAM HUU CHANH, NGUYEN DAT XUONG, & AZUM-GELADE, M.-C. (1971) Etude toxicologique de la formamide et de ses dérivés N-méthylés et N-éthylés. *Thérapie*, **26**: 409-424.

PHAM HUU CHANH, AZUM-GELADE, M.-C., NGUYEN VAN BAC, & NGUYEN DAT XUONG (1973) Cardiovascular activity of N,N-dimethylformamide. *Toxicology*, **1**: 135-142.

POIRIER, S.H., KNUTH, M.L., ANDERSON-BUCHOU, C.D., BROOKE, L.T., LIMA, A.R., & SHUBAT, P.J. (1986) Comparative toxicity of methanol and N,N-dimethylformamide to freshwater fish and invertebrates. *Bull. environ. Contam. Toxicol.*, **37**: 615-621.

POTTER, H.P. (1973) Dimethylformamide induced abdominal pain and liver injury. *Arch. environ. Health*, **27**: 340-341.

PURCHASE, I.F.H., LONGSTAFF, E., ASHBY, J., STYLES, J.A., ANDERSON, D., LEFEVRE, P.A., & WESTWOOD, F.R. (1978) An evaluation of six short-term tests for detecting organic chemical cancerogens. *Br. J. Cancer*, **37**: 873-903.

QIN, Y.H. & GUE, R.R. (1976) [Studies on the maximum allowalble concentration of dimethylformamide in surface water.] *J. Hyg. Res.*, **5**(2): 161-167 (in Chinese).

REBHUN, L.J. & SAWADA, N. (1969) Augmentation and dispersion of the *in vivo* mitotic apparatus of living marine eggs. *Protoplasma*, **68**: 1-22.

ROMADINA, E.S. (1975) [Direct action of microorganisms - one way of increasing the effectiveness of biological purification of waste waters.] In: Telitchenko, M., ed. *[Biological self-purification in water quality management: Proceedings of the All-Union Symposium on Sanitary Hydrobiology.]* Moscow, Nauka, pp. 110-112 (in Russian).

SALA, C., BERNABEO, F., COLOMBO, G., INVERNIZZI, E., & MENEGHEL, G. (1984) Dimethylformamide risk. An evaluation in the production of artificial organic leather. *Med. Lav.* **6**: 143-148.

SANOTSKY, I.V. & ULANOVA, I.P. (1975) *[Criteria for harmfulness in hygiene and toxicology for evaluation of hazards from chemical compounds.]* Moscow, Medizina, 372 pp (in Russian).

SANOTSKY, I.V., MURAVIEVA, S.I., ZAEVA, G.N., ANVAER, L., & SEMILETKINA, N.N. (1978) [Metabolism of dimethylformamide depending on the intensity of its action.] *Gig. Tr. prof. Zabol.*, **11**: 24-27 (in Russian).

SANSONE, E.B. & TEWARI, Y.B. (1978) The permeability of laboratory gloves to selected solvents. *Am. Ind. Hyg. Assoc. J.*, **39**(2): 169-174.

SANTA CRUZ, G. & CORPINO, P. (1978) [Preliminary morphological studies on acute experimental inhalation exposure in the rat.] *Boll. Soc. Ital. Biol. Sper.*, **54**: 1710-1717 (in Italian).

SANTA CRUZ, G. & MACCIONI, A. (1978) [Experimental study on dimethylformamide toxicity. Changes of the myocardium after prolonged inhalation treatment in the rat.] *Boll. Soc. Ital. Biol. Sper.*, **54**: 1717-1722 (in Italian).

SASAKI, S. (1978) The scientific aspects of the chemical substance control law in Japan. In: Hutzinger, O., Lelyveld, L.H., van, & Zoeteman, B.C.J., ed., *Aquatic pollutants: Transformation and biological effects*, Oxford, New York, Pergamon Press.

SAVOLAINEN, H. (1981) Dose-dependant effects of peroral dimethylformamide administration on rat brain. *Acta neuropathol.*, **53**: 249-252.

SCAILTEUR, V. (1984) *Contribution à l'étude de la relation toxicité-metabolisme de la dimethylformamide chez le rat*. Université Catholique de Louvain, 255 pp. (Thèse).

SCAILTEUR, V. & LAUWERYS, R. (1984a) *In vivo* and *in vitro* oxidative biotransformation of dimethylformamide in rat. *Chem.-biol. Interact.*, **50**: 327-337.

SCAILTEUR, V. & LAUWERYS, R. (1984b) *In vivo* metabolism of dimethylformamide and relationship to toxicity in the male rat. *Arch. Toxicol.*, **56**: 87-91.

SCAILTEUR, V. & LAUWERYS, R.R. (1987) Dimethylformamide (DMF) hepatotoxicity. *Toxicology*, **43**: 231-238.

SCAILTEUR, V., HOFFMANN, E., BUCHET, J.P., & LAUWERYS, R. (1984) Study on *in vivo* and *in vitro* metabolism of dimethylformamide in male and female rats. *Toxicology*, **29**: 222-234.

SCHEUFLER, H., VON, & FREYE, H.-A. (1975) [Embryotoxic and teratogenic effects of dimethylformamide.] *Dtsch. Gesundheitswes.*, **30**: 455-459 (in German).

SCHOTTEK, W. (1964) [Problems with the standardization of embryotoxic substances.] *Z. ärztl. Fortbild.*, **64**: 1158-1162 (in German).

SCHOTTEK, W. (1970) [Experimental dimethylformamide toxicity studies on experimental animals after repeated treatment.] *Acta. biol. med. Germ.*, **25**: 359-361 (in German).

References

SCHOTTEK, W. (1972) [Towards the problem of hygiene standardization of chemicals having embryotoxic action.] In: *Sanotsky, I.V., ed. [Hygiene standardization in study of remote effects of industrial substances.*] Moscow, Medizina, pp. 119-123 (in Russian).

SERRES, F.J., DE & ASHBY, J., ed. (1981) *Evaluation of short-term tests for carcinogens*, Amsterdam, Oxford, New York, Elsevier Science Publishers, 827 pp (Progress in Mutation Research, Vol. 1).

SHARKAWI, M. (1980) Inhibition of alcoholdehydrogenase by dimethylformamide and dimethylsulfoxide. *Toxicol. Lett.*, **4**: 493-497.

SHEVELEVA, G.A. & OSINA, S.A. (1973) [Experimental investigation of the embryotropic action of dimethylformamide.] In: [*The toxicology of new industrial chemicals.*] Moscow, Medizina, Vol. 13, pp. 75-82 (in Russian).

SHEVELEVA, G.A., STREKALOVA, E.E., & CHIRKOVA, E.M. (1979) [Study of the embryotropic, mutagenic, and gonadotropic effects of dimethylformamide after inhibition exposure.] In: [*The toxicology of new industrial chemicals.*] Moscow, Medizina, Vol. 15, pp. 21-25 (in Russian).

SHLYGINA, O.E. & NEMOLCHEV, V.M. (1981) [The use of radio-isotope methods in studies of acute poisoning with dimethylformamide.] In: [*Proceedings of the Moscow Scientific Research Institute of First Aid.*] Moscow, Medizina, Vol. 45: 130-132 (in Russian).

SHUBAT, P.J., POIRIER, S.H., KNUTH, M.L., & BROOKE, L.T. (1982) Acute toxicity of tetrachloroethylene and tetrachloroethylene with dimethylformamide to rainbow trout, *Salmo gairdneri. Bull. environ. Contam. Toxicol.*, **28**: 7-10.

SICKLES, J.E., WRIGHT, R.S., SUTCLIFFE, C.R., BLAKARD, A.L., & DAYTON, D.P. (1980) Smog chamber studies of the reactivity of volatile organic compounds. In: *Proceedings of the 73rd Annual Meeting of the Air Pollution Control Association* (Paper 80-50.1).

STOCKLEY, I.H. (1983) Drugs, foods, and environmental chemical agents which can initiate Antabuse-like reactions with alcohol. *Pharmacol. Interact.*, **4**: 12-16.

STRANSKY, V. (1986) The determination of *N,N*-dimethylformamide in working atmosphere by the method of gas chromatography after sampling on activated charcoal. *Prac. Lek.*, **38**: 15-19.

STULA, E.F. & KRAUSS, W.C. (1977) Embryotoxicity in rats and rabbits from cutaneous application of amide type solvents and substituted ureas. *Toxicol. appl. Pharmacol.*, **41**: 35-55.

TACCOLA, A., CATENACCI, G., & BARUFFINI, A. (1981) Cardiotoxicity of dimethylformamide (DMF). Electrocardiographic findings and continuous electrocardiographic monitoring. *G. Ital. Med. Lav.*, **3**: 149-151.

TANAKA, K.I. (1971) Toxicity of dimethylformamide (DMF) to the young female rat. *Int. Arch. Arbeitsmed.*, **28**: 98-105.

TANAKA, K.I. & UTSUNOMIYA, T. (1982) [The toxicity of N,N-dimethylformamide (DMF).] *Jpn. J. ind. Health*, **24**: 3-12 (in Japanese).

THIERSCH, J.E. (1962) Effects of acetamides and formamides on the rat litter *in utero*. *J. Reprod. Fertil.*, **4**: 220.

TOLOT, F., DROIN, M., & GENEVOIS, J. (1958) Intoxication par la diméthylformamide. *Arch. Mal. prof.*, **19**: 602-606.

TOLOT, F., ARCADIO, F., LENGLET, J.-P., & ROCHE, L. (1968) Intoxication par la diméthylformamide. *Arch. Mal. prof.*, **29**: 714-717.

TOMASINI, M., TODARO, A., PIAZZONI, M., & PERUZZO, G.F. (1983) [Pathology due to dimethylformamide. Observation of 14 cases.] *Med. Lav.*, **74**: 217-220 (in Italian).

TONOGAI, Y., OGAWA, S., ITO, Y., & IWAIDA, M. (1982) Actual survey on TLM (median tolerance limit) values of environmental pollutants, especially on amines, nitriles, aromatic nitrogen compounds and artificial dyes. *J. toxicol. Sci.*, **7**: 193-203.

UNGAR, H., SULLMAN, S.F., & ZUCKERMAN, A.J. (1976) Acute and protracted changes in the liver of Syrian hamsters induced by a single dose of aflatoxin B_1. Observations on pathological effects of the solvent dimethylformamide. *Br. J. exp. Pathol.*, **57**: 157- 164.

US EPA (1986) *Health and environmental effects profile for N,N-dimethylformamide*. Cincinnati, Ohio, US Environmental Protection Agency, Health and Environmental Assessment, Environment Criteria and Assessment Office, 106 pp (Unpublished data).

US NIOSH (1978) *Occupational health guideline for dimethylformamide*, Cincinnati, Ohio, US National Institute for Occupational Safety and Health, 5 pp.

US NIOSH (1977) *Manual of analytical methods*, Cincinnati, Ohio, US National Institute for Occupational Safety and Health, Vol. 3 (No. S-255).

WAHLBERG, J.E. & BOMAN, A. (1979) Comparative percutaneous toxicity of ten industrial solvents in the guinea-pig. *Scand. J. Work Environ. Health*, **5**: 345-351.

WALRATH, J., FAYERWEATHER, M.P.H., & GILBY, C.I.H. (1988) *A case-control study of cancer among Du Pont employees with potential for exposure to dimethylformamide*, Wilmington, Delaware, E.I. Du Pont de Nemours Co. (Unpublished report).

References

WEISS, G. (1971) [Industrial dimethylformamide intoxication and the question of its recognition as an occupational disease.] *Zbl. Arbeitsmed.*, **11**: 345-346 (in German).

WELWARD, L. & HALAMA, D. (1978) Influence of anti-microbial agents on contamination and chlorotetracycline production. *Folia microbiol.*, **23**: 12-17.

WICAROVA, O. & DADAK, O. (1981) [Urinary N-methylformamide levels in persons exposed to dimethylformamide vapour.] *Prac. Lek.*, **33**: 42-46 (in Czech).

WILES, J.S. & NARCISSE, J.K., Jr (1971) The acute toxicity of dimethylformamides in several animal species. *Am. Ind. Hyg. Assoc. J.*, **32**: 539-545.

WILSON, H.K. & OTTLEY, T.W. (1981) The use of a transportable mass spectrometer for the direct measurement of industrial solvents in breath. *Biomed. mass. Spectrom.*, **8**: 606-610.

YONEMOTO, J. & SUZUKI, S. (1980) Relation of exposure to dimethylformamide vapour and the metabolite, methylformamide, in urine of workers. *Int. Arch. occup. environ. Health*, **46**: 159-165.

RESUME ET EVALUATION, CONCLUSIONS, RECOMMANDATIONS

1. Résumé et évaluation

1.1 Propriétés générales

Le N,N-diméthylformamide (diméthylformamide, DMF, CSA 68-12-1) est un solvant organique qui est produit en grandes quantités dans l'ensemble du monde. On l'utilise dans l'industrie chimique comme solvant, comme produit intermédiaire et comme additif. Le DMF est un liquide incolore d'odeur légère mais désagréable qui, néanmoins, est insuffisante pour attirer l'attention. Il est généralement stable mais il peut entraîner des incendies et des explosions par contact avec des oxydants forts, des halogènes, des dérivés alkylaluminiques ou des hydrocarbures halogénés (en particulier combinés à des métaux). Le DMF est entièrement miscible à l'eau et à la plupart des solvants organiques. Sa tension de vapeur est relativement faible.

Du point de vue analytique, on a recours à la chromatographie en phase gazeuse.

1.2 Transport, distribution, et transformation dans l'environnement

Le DMF est stable dans l'air ambiant mais il peut subir une décomposition microbienne et algaire dans l'eau. Les microorganismes adaptés et les boues activées assurent une biodégradation efficace du DMF. Etant soluble dans l'eau en toutes proportions, le DMF est très mobile dans les sols et il ne devrait pas s'accumuler dans la chaîne alimentaire.

1.3 Concentration dans l'environnement et exposition humaine

Le DMF n'existe pas à l'état naturel. On ne possède que peu de données sur sa concentration dans l'environnement ou sur l'exposition de la population générale. Dans l'air de zones résidentielles situées à proximité d'installations industrielles, on a trouvé des concentrations allant de 0,02 à 0,12 mg/m^3. Il est rare qu'on décèle la présence de DMF dans l'eau des bassins fluviaux très industrialisés et encore, les concentrations ne dépassent pas 0,01 mg/litre.

Résumé et évaluation, conclusions, recommandations

On ne possède pas de données sur la concentration du DMF dans le sol, les végétaux, la faune sauvage et les produits alimentaires.

L'exposition professionnelle se produit par contact cutané avec le liquide ou la vapeur ou par inhalation de la vapeur. On a décelé des concentrations de 3 à 86 mg/m^3 dans l'air avec des maxima allant jusqu'à 600 mg/m^3, au cours de travaux de réparation ou d'entretien de machines. Dans quelques cas exceptionnels, des concentrations allant jusqu'à 4500 mg/m^3 ont été signalées.

1.4 Cinétique et métabolisme

Des quantités toxiques de DMF peuvent être absorbées par inhalation ou pénétration percutanée. Une fois absorbé, le DMF se distribue de façon uniforme dans l'organisme. Sa métabolisation a lieu principalement dans le foie sous l'action des enzymes microsomiales. Chez l'animal et l'homme, le principal produit de la biotransformation du DMF est le *N*-hydroxyméthyl-*N*-méthylformamide (DMF-OH). Au cours de l'analyse par chromatographie en phase gazeuse, ce métabolite est transformé en *N*-méthylformamide (NMF) qui est lui-même (ainsi que le *N*-hydroxyméthyl et le formamide) un métabolite mineur du DMF. Par conséquent, lorsqu'on procède à des études métaboliques et que l'on effectue la surveillance biologique du DMF, les concentrations urinaires de métabolites sont mesurées et exprimées en NMF, même si le DMF-OH en est le constituant essentiel. Le dosage du NMF/DMF-OH dans les urines peut donner une bonne indication biologique de l'exposition totale au DMF.

Chez l'animal d'expérience, on a montré que le mécanisme de métabolisation du DMF se sature lorsque l'exposition est intense, le DMF jouant le rôle de rétroinhibiteur de son propre métabolisme à concentration très élevée.

Il y a interaction métabolique entre le DMF et l'éthanol.

1.5 Effets sur les êtres vivant dans leur milieu naturel

On n'a pas très bien étudié les effets du DMF sur l'environnement. Il semble que sa toxicité pour les organismes aquatiques soit faible.

1.6 Effets sur les animaux d'expérience et les systèmes d'épreuve in vitro

Le DMF présente pour diverses espèces une faible toxicité aiguë (chez le rat la DL_{50} par voie orale est d'environ 3000 mg/kg, la DL_{50} dermique d'environ 5000 mg/kg et la CL_{50} par inhalation à peu près égale à 10 000 mg/m^3). Il est légèrement à modérément irritant pour la peau et les yeux. D'après une étude sur des cobayes, il ne semble pas doté de pouvoir sensibilisateur. Le DMF peut faciliter l'absorption percutanée d'autres substances chimiques.

Chez l'animal d'expérience, l'exposition au DMF, quelle que soit la voie de pénétration, peut provoquer des lésions hépatiques qui dépendent de la dose. Lorsque l'exposition cesse, on a pu constater qu'il y avait régénération des tissus. Certaines études ont également permis d'observer des signes de toxicité au niveau du myocarde et des reins.

On n'a pas constaté de toxicité pour les testicules ou les ovaires, ni observé d'effets sur la fécondité chez le rat. Chez le rat, la souris et le lapin, le DMF s'est révélé embryotoxique et faiblement tératogène. C'est le lapin qui est l'espèce la plus sensible à l'exposition respiratoire: des effets tératogènes ont été observés à partir de 1350 mg/m^3 (450 ppm), aucun effet n'étant constaté à 450 mg/m^3 (150 ppm). Après exposition de la peau, certaines études ont mis en évidence de très rares effets embryotoxiques et tératogènes à des doses journalières comprises entre 100 et 400 mg/kg.

De nombreuses épreuves à court terme à la recherche d'effets génétiques et anomalies de ce genre ont montré que le DMF était en général inactif tant *in vitro* qu'*in vivo*.

Aucune étude convenable de cancérogénicité à long terme sur animaux de laboratoire n'est décrite dans la littérature.

Résumé et évaluation, conclusions, recommandations

1.7 Effets sur l'homme

Aucun effet indésirable sur la population dans son ensemble n'a été nettement mis en évidence.

On a fait état d'irritation cutanée et de conjonctivites après contact direct avec du DMF.

Après exposition accidentelle à de fortes concentrations de DMF, on note dans les 48h. des douleurs abdominales, des nausées, des étourdissements et de la fatigue. La fonction hépatique peut être perturbée et on a signalé des modifications de la tension artérielle, une tachycardie et des anomalies du tracé électrocardiographique. En général la récupération est totale.

Après des expositions réitérées sur une longue période, on observe des symptômes tels que céphalées, perte d'appétit et fatigue. Des signes biochimiques d'insuffisance hépatique peuvent également s'observer. Des lésions hépatiques n'apparaissent, semble-t-il, qu'à partir d'une exposition de l'ordre de 30 mg/m^3, en l'absence de contact cutané. Cette concentration atmosphérique correspond à environ 40 mg de NMF/DMF-OH par gramme de créatinine dans un échantillon d'urine prélevé à la fin du poste de travail.

Même à des concentrations inférieures à 30 mg/m^3, l'exposition au DMF peut causer une intolérance à l'alcool dont les symptômes peuvent consister en rougeur soudaine de la face, sensation de constriction thoracique et étourdissements, quelques fois accompagnés de nausées et de dyspnée. Ces symptômes durent de 2 à 4 heures et disparaissent spontanément.

On possède des preuves limitées d'une activité cancérogène du DMF pour l'homme. C'est ainsi qu'une étude a fait état d'un accroissement de l'incidence des tumeurs du testicule après exposition à du DMF, tandis qu'une autre étude a révélé une incidence tumorale accrue au niveau de la cavité buccale et du pharynx, mais pas au niveau des testicules.

Deux études peu détaillées font état d'un accroissement de la fréquence des avortements chez des femmes exposées à du DMF, entre autres substances chimiques.

2. Conclusions

1. Compte tenu de ses usages actuels, la population dans son ensemble n'est probablement que très peu exposée au DMF.

2. Le DMF est facilement résorbé au niveau de la peau et des voies respiratoires. Le dosage dans les urines du NMF/DMF-OH constitue un moyen utile pour évaluer la quantité totale de DMF absorbé.

3. Le risque de lésions hépatiques est faible si la concentration du DMF dans l'air ambiant est maintenue en dessous de 30 mg/m^3 et qu'il n'y a pas de contact cutané. La valeur correspondante de la teneur des urines en NMF/DMF-OH à la fin du poste de travail a été fixée provisoirement à 40 mg/g de créatinine.

4. Le DMF est embryotoxique et faiblement tératogène pour le rat, la souris et le lapin.

5. Il existe des preuves limitées d'une cancérogénicité du DMF pour l'homme.

6. D'après les données dont on dispose, le DMF est peu toxique pour l'environnement. Il est peu probable qu'il donne lieu à une bioaccumulation.

3. Recommandations

3.1 Précautions à prendre pour la manipulation

1. Maintenir la concentration atmosphérique au-dessous de 30 mg/m^3 et éviter le contact avec la peau.

2. Surveiller la concentration urinaire de NMF/DMF-OH qui indique l'exposition totale et la maintenir en-dessous de 40 mg de NMF/g de créatinine dans les échantillons prélevés à la fin du poste de travail. Si la concentration

Résumé et évaluation, conclusions, recommandations

dépasse cette valeur, prendre les mesures nécessaires pour réduire l'exposition.

3.2 Recherches à effectuer

1. Etudier les effets cancérogènes possibles du DMF chez l'homme, par des études sur des populations humaines et des animaux d'expérience.

2. Il faudrait disposer de données plus complètes sur la possibilité d'extrapoler à l'homme les résultats des études d'embryotoxicité et de tératogénicité effectuées sur l'animal. Il serait bon d'étudier la cinétique comparée du DMF chez l'homme et l'animal.

3. Davantage de données sont nécessaires sur le mode d'action et l'activité relative des métabolites du DMF chez l'homme et l'animal.

4. Il faudrait affiner les relations entre a) les concentrations en métabolites urinaires et les taux d'exposition atmosphérique (en l'absence de contact cutané), et b) la dose totale absorbée par toutes les voies possibles (indiquée par la concentration en NMF urinaire à la fin du poste de travail) et l'absence d'hépatotoxicité.

RESUMEN Y EVALUACION, CONCLUSIONES, RECOMENDACIONES

1. Resumen y evaluación

1.1 Propiedades generales

La *N,N*-dimetilformamida (dimetilformamida, DMF, CAS 68-12-2) es un disolvente orgánico que se produce en grandes cantidades en todo el mundo. Se utiliza en la industria química como disolvente, compuesto intermedio y aditivo. La DMF es un líquido incoloro con un ligero olor desagradable que, no obstante, tiene escasas propiedades de alerta. Es generalmente estable, pero cuando entra en contacto con oxidantes fuertes, halógenos, alquilaluminio o hidrocarburos halogenados (especialmente en combinación con metales), puede prenderse y provocar explosiones. La DMF es totalmente miscible con el agua y la mayoría de los disolventes orgánicos. Su presión de vapor es relativamente baja.

Existen procedimientos de cromatografía de gases para la determinación de la DMF.

1.2 Transporte, distribución y transformación en el medio ambiente

Aunque la DMF es estable en el aire, puede ser objeto en el agua de degradación por microbios y algas. Los microorganismos adaptados y los fangos activados biodegradan la DMF de modo eficiente. A consecuencia de su solubilidad total en el agua, la DMF se desplaza fácilmente en el suelo y no es de esperar que se acumule en la cadena alimentaria.

1.3 Niveles medioambientales y exposición humana

La DMF no aparece en la naturaleza. Se dispone de pocos datos relativos a los niveles medioambientales o a la exposición de la población general a la DMF. En zonas residenciales cercanas a centros industriales se han medido concentraciones atmosféricas de 0,02-0,12 mg/m^3. Se ha detectado muy raras veces en las aguas de cuencas fluviales muy industrializadas, y en esos casos sólo en concentraciones inferiores a 0,01 mg/litro.

No se dispone de datos relativos a los niveles de DMF en el suelo, los vegetales, los animales silvestres ni los alimentos.

La exposición profesional se produce por contacto cutáneo con la DMF en forma líquida y de vapor, y por la inhalación de vapores. Se han detectado concentraciones de 3-86 mg/m^3 de aire, con valores máximos de hasta 600 mg/m^3, durante las operaciones de reparación o de mantenimiento de máquinas. En condiciones muy especiales, se han registrado concentraciones de hasta 4500 mg/m^3.

1.4 Cinética y metabolismo

Pueden absorberse cantidades tóxicas de DMF por inhalación y a través de la piel. La DMF absorbida se distribuye uniformemente. La transformación metabólica de la DMF tiene lugar principalmente en el hígado, con el concurso de sistemas de enzimas microsómicas. En los animales y el ser humano, el producto principal de la biotransformación de la DMF es la *N*-hidroximetil-*N*-metilformamida (DMF-OH). Este metabolito principal se convierte durante el análisis con cromatografía de gases en *N*-metilformamida, que es a su vez (junto con la *N*-hidroximetilformamida y la formamida) uno de los metabolitos secundarios. Así pues, en los estudios metabólicos y para el monitoreo biológico, las concentraciones de metabolitos en la orina se miden y expresan en forma de NMF, aunque la DMF-OH sea el contribuyente principal a esa concentración. El análisis de la NMF/DMF-OH en la orina puede ser un indicador biológico adecuado de la exposición total a la DMF.

En los animales de experimentación, se ha demostrado que el metabolismo de la DMF se satura a niveles de exposición elevados y que, a niveles muy elevados, la DMF inhibe su propio metabolismo.

Se produce interacción metabólica entre la DMF y el etanol.

1.5 Efectos en los organismos del medio ambiente

No se han estudiado bien los efectos de la DMF en el medio ambiente. La toxicidad para los organismos acuáticos parece baja.

1.6 Efectos en los animales de experimentación y en sistemas de ensayo in vitro

La toxicidad aguda de la DMF en diversas especies es baja (en ratas, la DL_{50} es de unos 3000 mg/kg, la DL_{50} cutánea es de aproximadamente 5000 mg/kg, y la LC_{50} por inhalación es de unos 10 000 mg/m^3. Su capacidad de irritación de la piel y los ojos es entre ligera y moderada. En un estudio realizado con cobayas no hubo indicación alguna de potencial de sensibilización. La DMF puede facilitar la absorción de otras sustancias químicas a través de la piel.

La exposición de animales de experimentación a la DMF por todas las vías de exposición puede provocar lesiones hepáticas dependientes de la dosis. Se ha demostrado que se produce regeneración al cesar la exposición. En algunos estudios se han descrito asimismo síntomas de toxicidad en el miocardio y el riñón.

No se ha demostrado que la DMF sea tóxica para el testículo ni para el ovario de la rata, ni se han observado efectos en la fecundidad. Se ha descubierto que la DMF es embriotóxica y ligeramente teratogénica en la rata, el ratón y el conejo. El conejo parece ser la especie más sensible a la exposición por inhalación: se observaron efectos teratogénicos a partir de 1350 mg/m^3 (450 ppm), pero no a 450 mg/m^3 (150 ppm). Tras la exposición cutánea, en algunos estudios se observó una incidencia muy baja de efectos embriotóxicos y teratogénicos con dosis que variaron entre 100 y 400 mg/kg al día.

En una amplia serie de ensayos a corto plazo en busca de efectos genéticos y otros afines se encontró que, en general, la DMF es inactiva, tanto *in vitro* como *in vivo*.

No se han comunicado estudios suficientes sobre carcinogenicidad a largo plazo en animales de experimentación.

1.7 Efectos en el ser humano

No se ha demostrado claramente la existencia de efectos adversos de la DMF en la población general.

Se han comunicado casos de irritación cutánea y conjuntivitis tras el contacto directo con DMF.

Al cabo de 48 horas de la exposición accidental a niveles elevados de DMF, aparecen dolores abdominales, náuseas, vómitos, mareos y fatiga. La función hepática puede alterarse y se han notificado casos de cambios en la tensión arterial, taquicardia y anomalías electroencefalográficas. Por lo general, la recuperación es completa.

Después de una exposición repetida y a largo plazo, aparecen síntomas como dolor de cabeza, pérdida de apetito y fatiga. Pueden observarse signos de disfunción hepática. Las lesiones hepáticas parecen producirse sólo cuando el nivel de exposición a la DMF pasa de 30 mg/m^3, en ausencia de contacto cutáneo. Ese nivel en el aire corresponde a aproximadamente 40 mg de NMF/DMF-OH/creatinina en una muestra de orina tomada después del turno de trabajo.

La exposición a la DMF, incluso en concentraciones inferiores a 30 mg/m^3, puede provocar intolerancia al alcohol. Entre los síntomas pueden presentarse un acaloramiento facial repentino, opresión en el pecho y mareos, a veces acompañados de náuseas y disnea. Duran entre 2 y 4 h y desaparecen espontáneamente.

Existen pruebas limitadas de que la DMF es carcinogénica para el ser humano. En un estudio se comunicó una incidencia mayor de tumores testiculares, mientras que en otro se observó una incidencia mayor de tumores de la cavidad oral y la faringe, pero no del testículo.

En dos estudios, que comunican pocos pormenores, se observó una frecuencia mayor de abortos espontáneos en mujeres expuestas a la DMF, entre otras sustancias químicas.

2. Conclusiones

1. Dados los usos actuales de la DMF, la exposición de la población general es probablemente muy baja.

2. La DMF se absorbe fácilmente a través de la piel además de por inhalación. La determinación de la NMF/DMF-OH en la orina

es un medio muy útil de estimar la cantidad total de DMF absorbida.

3. El riesgo de lesión hepática es reducido si el nivel de DMF en el aire se mantiene por debajo de 30 mg/m^3 y no hay contacto cutáneo. Un valor provisional para el nivel correspondiente de NMF/DMF-OH en la orina en una muestra tomada después del turno de trabajo es 40 mg/g de creatinina.

4. La DMF es embriotóxica y ligeramente teratogénica en la rata, el ratón y el conejo.

5. Existen pruebas limitadas de la carcinogenicidad de la DMF para el ser humano.

6. Los datos disponibles indican que tiene una baja toxicidad ambiental. Es poco probable que se produzca bioacumulación.

3. Recomendaciones

3.1 Manipulación sin riesgos

1. Las concentraciones en el aire deben mantenerse por debajo de 30 mg/m^3 y debe evitarse el contacto con la piel.

2. La NMF/DMF-OH en la orina, como índice de la exposición total, debe vigilarse y mantenerse por debajo de 40 mg de NMF/g de creatinina en muestras tomadas después del turno de trabajo. Si se sobrepasa ese nivel, deben adoptarse medidas para disminuir la exposición.

3.2 Nuevas investigaciones

1. Los posibles efectos carcinogénicos del DMF en el ser humano deben investigarse mediante estudios en animales de experimentación y poblaciones humanas.

2. Se necesita más información para extrapolar de los estudios en animales al ser humano los datos sobre embriotoxicidad y

teratogenicidad de la DMF. La comparación de la cinética de la DMF en el ser humano y en los animales sería muy útil.

3. Se necesita más información sobre los mecanismos de acción y la potencia relativa de los metabolitos de la DMF en animales y en el ser humano.

4. Deben afinarse las relaciones entre a) las concentraciones de metabolitos en la orina y los niveles de exposición en la atmósfera (en ausencia de contacto cutáneo), y b) la dosis total recibida por todas las vías (indicada por los niveles de NMF en la orina después del trabajo) y la ausencia de hepatotoxicidad.

www.ingramcontent.com/pod-product-compliance
Ingram Content Group UK Ltd.
Pitfield, Milton Keynes, MK11 3LW, UK
UKHW021310180426
11947UKWH00015B/1132